NURSING PRINCIPLES

Nursing Principles

A GUIDE FOR PRACTICE

JAN SNOWBALL
BA, SRN, RCNT, RNT
Senior Tutor
School of Nursing
Oxford

WENDY H. GREEN
SRN, RNT, ONC, OHNC,
Teaching Certificate, ACE
Tutor
Clinical Practice Development
School of Nursing
Oxford

SECOND EDITION

Blackwell Scientific Publications

OXFORD LONDON EDINBURGH

BOSTON PALO ALTO MELBOURNE

First edition © by
Oxfordshire Health Authority
Second edition © by
Blackwell Scientific Publications
Editorial offices:
Osney Mead, Oxford OX2 0EL
 (*Orders*: Tel. 0865 240201)
8 John Street, London WC1N 2ES
23 Ainslie Place, Edinburgh EH3 6AJ
52 Beacon Street, Boston
 Massachusetts 02108, USA
667 Lytton Avenue, Palo Alto
 California 94301, USA
107 Barry Street, Carlton
 Victoria 3053, Australia

First published 1986
Second edition 1987

Photoset by Enset (Photosetting),
Midsomer Norton, Bath, Avon
Printed and bound
in Great Britain

DISTRIBUTORS

USA
 Year Book Medical Publishers
 35 East Wacker Drive
 Chicago, Illinois 60601
 (*Orders*: Tel. 312 726-9733)

Canada
 The C.V. Mosby Company
 5240 Finch Avenue East
 Scarborough, Ontario
 (*Orders*: Tel. 416-298-1588)

Australia
 Blackwell Scientific Publications
 (Australia) Pty Ltd
 107 Barry Street
 Carlton, Victoria 3053
 (*Orders*: Tel. (03) 347 0300)

British Library
Cataloguing in Publication Data

Snowball, Jan
 Nursing principles: a guide for
 practice.
 —2nd ed.
 1. Nursing
 I. Title II. Green, Wendy H.
 610.73   RT41

ISBN 0-632-01812-7

Contents

Preface

In the past, Oxford, like most other nurse teaching hospitals in the country, possessed a Procedure Committee, the role of which was to formulate policy statements regarding nursing skills. These statements dictated trolley settings and a step-by-step approach which was to be followed by every nurse undertaking that particular task. In fact these procedures provided the wherewithal to enable 'task orientated care' to continue. The 'procedures' ranged from the common place (e.g. bedbathing, mouth care, care of the hair) to the very specialized (e.g. catheterization of the umbilicus of the newborn, application of plaster of paris splint).

In 1983 Oxfordshire Health Authority, recognizing recent advances in nursing, replaced the Procedure Committee with the Nursing Practices Committee.

The terms of reference for this committee are:

1 To provide advice to the Authority and its Nursing Officer on matters concerning professional nursing practice and on any matters referred to it by the Authority or its Nursing Officer.

2 To convene standards groups to advise on major areas of nursing practice, taking into account practice developments and research, and to submit recommendations to the Nursing Policy Group.

3 To produce guidelines for qualified nurses on new nursing work, and to submit recommendations to the Nursing Policy Group.

4 To produce guidelines for nurses in training and their supervisors, on the English National Board's syllabi.

In response to Item 4 of the terms of reference, the Committee sought a new framework from which nurses in training, and qualified nurses, could derive the actions they needed to take. A small booklet *Nursing Principles—a guide for practice* evolved. This was carefully tested by students, their teachers, and qualified clinical staff. It was so well received, both inside and outside the district, that this expanded, and updated version is now offered.

The Nursing Practices Committee was unanimous in agreeing that practice guidelines should be in terms of principles, since a task orientated approach to patient care meant that each nurse in a ward area performed those tasks or procedures for all the patients for whom they were prescribed. Any one patient was therefore cared for by many nurses, who took responsibility for the several parts of the total care given. Within this framework it was difficult for the patient to establish a relationship with any one nurse, or indeed to be assured of being nursed as an individual. Care of the patient was very fragmented, the only person likely to see the 'whole picture' with regard to any one patient, being the person in charge of the ward.

Unrelated techniques and routines cannot teach the true value of patient centred care. The adoption of a holistic framework guiding curriculum design in the School of Nursing, together with the expectations of the English National Board, outlined in the 1983 consultation paper, plus the fact that new nursing knowledge, derived from research, arises almost daily, demonstrates that the logical approach is to outline the principles of nursing care, from which the method can be derived and learnt alongside a role model—a qualified nurse who is capable of adjusting care independently and critically appraising each step of the process.

In order to identify principles of nursing practice, activities of daily living have been used as a framework for reference in Part I. Part II carries the application further and expands on those nursing skills which are not specifically related to activities of daily living but are an essential component of patient care. Where appropriate, guidelines for specific aspects of nursing practice, commonly used throughout the health district have been included in the text. In Part III some of the professional/organizational issues which may have a direct effect on nursing practice have been included.

The book is used by teachers in the School of Nursing, supplemented by other substantial texts, for introducing and teaching nursing principles in lecture and seminar work before, and as, the student applies the principles to the nursing of patients.

It has been made available to all clinical staff so that they know the principles the students have been taught and are able to use the same principles in their teaching, supervision and assessment of students.

A book of nursing principles does not deny the need for specialist procedures such as those referred to earlier, e.g. catheterization of the umbilicus of the newborn. However, it is believed that these specialist procedures, which may change frequently, should be drawn up by the clinical staff involved, and held locally in the specialist area.

We are conscious that the idea is experimental and that as people use the book they will have suggestions for how it can be improved and used in different ways; we would appreciate comments.

January 1987   *Jan Snowball, Wendy Green*

In using this book it should be noted that each principle has been highlighted in a box, and the statements following are derived from that principle.

Acknowledgements

A number of people have contributed to the production of this book, and we would like to express our gratitude to them.

Thanks are due to Jane Hathaway, Sue Rae, Karen Wilson, Jenny Burgess and Catherine Welch, who not only contributed clinical expertise, but also moral support when motivation and ideas flagged.

Thanks are also due to members of the Nursing Practices Committee of the Oxfordshire Health Authority for the support and information offered throughout the time of writing the book; and clinical staff and nurse teachers who introduced students to concepts embodied in the book, and who contributed suggestions on content, on the basis of this work.

A word of thanks is due to Barbara Vaughan, Senior Tutor, Clinical Practice Development Team, Oxford, who sustained our effort through constant encouragement, critical appraisal and friendship.

Introduction to
the Concept of Health

Health has been defined by the World Health Organization as:
> 'a state of complete mental, physical and social well-being, and
> not merely the absence of disease or infirmity.'

Some have suggested that complete health may be an unrealistic
expectation for every individual, and have therefore produced
modified definitions, for example:
> 'the enjoyment of the highest attainable standard of health is one
> of the fundamental rights of every human being, without
> distinction of race, religion, political belief, economic or social
> conditon.'

People can be viewed as holistic beings, whose biology, psychology, social and cultural inheritance are inextricably linked. They
constantly interact and react within a changing environment, using
innate and aquired coping mechanisms, and this dynamic interaction
is what makes each individual unique. Health depends on the ability
to cope with external and internal change, and on the unique perception of what health (and illness) mean.

Achieving maximal health for an individual requires the fostering
of psychological, social, and physical homeostasis. This has been
defined as the maintenance of a state of equilibrium within the body,
despite varying conditions and situations, and can only be satisfac-
torily maintained when psychological, social and physical needs are
met.

Need has been defined as 'the want of something which one
cannot well do without', or 'a state that requires relief'. One way to
view the concept of need is to take the theory of a hierarchy of needs,
as developed by Abraham Maslow.

The hierarchy comprises five levels of need, in priority sequence.
According to Maslow's theory, the ability to satisfy higher needs, and
ultimately achieve ones full potential, self-actualization, can only
occur when more basic needs are met. At any level of the hierarchy,
unmet need may result in fluctuations in the health of the individual.

Factors which may influence need, and thus health, include:

(i) biological
- innate genetic potential
- maturational and ageing processes

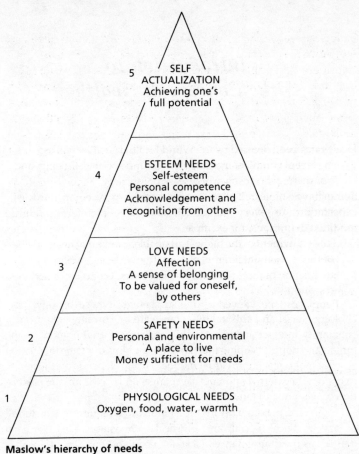

Maslow's hierarchy of needs

- physiological changes produced in interactions with the environment

(ii) psychological
- the emotional environment in which the individual lives
- interactions encountered
- coping mechanisms possessed

(iii) social
- the lifestyle chosen or available to the individual, for example in terms of, occupation, income, education, life-pattern
- societal expectations of living standards, and health

On any given occasion one unmet need, at any level, may supercede all others; at other times changes in need may appear inextricably linked.

Life transitions are typically times when psychological, social and biological needs change, and these are times when the health of the individual may become particularly susceptible to fluctuations. Some transitions can be anticipated, such as those of adolescence, marriage, or retirement, but others may be unexpected, such as the inability to find employment, redundancy or the untimely death of a loved one. Some transitions may have positive effects on the health of the individual, whilst others may result in more negative effects—all however, produce the stress of change and the need for readjustment, which, of itself, may affect health.

Transition also occurs on a wider societal scale, and may have just as much effect on individual health as the personal life history. The incidence of disease, for example, constantly changes, as does medical and technological advancement. Catastrophes such as war, famine, and earthquake affect many parts of the world. Societal aspirations for health and health services fluctuate, thus the demands made of the individual and society alter in terms of responsibility for maintaining health.

In recent years, in the Western world, health has assumed a more positive meaning—it is now no longer considered to be simply the absence of disease. Society now expects that the promotion and maintenance of health will become a high priority for each individual, as well as the focus of the health services. There is an implicit expectation that the health care organizations will be provided to:

(i) promote health

(ii) detect failing health at an early stage

(iii) initiate prompt treatment of disease, to limit morbidity and mortality.

These demands are largely met by:

(i) Primary health care services—the point of entry into the health care system, comprising all the helping agencies which people encounter in their own community: for example, general practitioners, health visitors, voluntary organizations. All provide education for the promotion and maintenance of health.

(ii) Secondary health care services—the support services providing for early detection of failing health, and early treatment: for example, hospital inpatient services. Here too the educational component exists.

(iii) Tertiary health care services—those that support individuals as they come to terms with health problems which may persist throughout life, and help to restore them to maximal individual health: for example, rehabilitation units for spinal injury patients.

An integrated policy is essential, which holds optimal health, rather than illness, to be the focus of care.

Societal expectations also influence demands on nursing for the future. Nursing, with its unique focus on basic human needs, can help to promote wellness, and to maintain and restore health. The success of nursing actions for health can be increased through knowledge, understanding, and a preparation for change in the light of the latest developments and aspirations.

Further reading

Maslow A.H. (1954) *Motivation and Personality*. Harper, New York.
World Health Organization (1948) *Constitution of WHO*, April 7. Geneva.

Introduction to the
Principles of Nursing Practice

Nursing is a dynamic profession which demands a strong sense of commitment and responsibility from the individual. The scope of professional nursing practice includes a much broader range of activities than is represented in the traditional image of the nurse. Although the nurse still performs many of the time-honoured functions in caring for the sick, the role has to expand and change to remain current with modern trends.

The nursing profession's concern, to maintain the quality of its service in the light of changing practice, constitutes the heart of its responsibility to the public. In order to guarantee that the quality of service is maintained, optimal standards of nursing practice are recognized as essential as a reassurance both for the public and the profession itself. Embodied in the need for high standards of nursing practice is the growing awareness of the accountability of nurses to the public they serve.

In recognition of the importance of standards of professional practice and the need to guarantee quality of service, the Nursing Service and School of Nursing for Oxfordshire have formulated a set of basic beliefs in respect of the patients cared for and the nursing service offered.

The patient/client

We believe that all patients are unique individuals with physical, spiritual, social and emotional needs. They are the centre of our entire nursing focus and have the right to considerate, honest and respectful care. We are aware also that the patient may be part of a family unit which, when possible and appropriate, should be included in the planning, implementation and education process.

The nurse

We believe that patients are best served by nurses who clearly understand the nature of professional nursing practice and who accept the responsibility of practising in a professional way. We recognize that nurses should be helped and supported in developing their professional practice, but maintaining professional competence is seen as the individual's responsibility. Similarly she is seen as having a personal responsibility to give instruction and guidance to peers and subordinates within her area of clinical expertise. To ensure the nurse fulfils the requirements of professional practice she should have regular opportunities to review her progress formally and to plan her development with her senior nursing manager.

Health care teams

The nurse cannot work in isolation, but rather she functions as a member of the health care team each of whom contributes special expertise in the care of the patient. It is important that all members have some idea of the contribution that others make in order to work co-operatively and have realistic expectations of their roles or responsibilities. As nursing is the only discipline that offers a continuous service, one of its major functions is the co-ordination of other team members and feedback to them of information.

Nursing

We believe that a critical component of delivering care is the use of the Nursing Process with a problem-solving approach. This approach could develop into a system of primary nursing where an individual registered nurse is responsible and accountable for a patient's nursing and is actively involved throughout his need for nursing.

Any guidance on nursing practice must be in terms of basic knowledge and skills upon which the practitioner can develop her own expertise. If we therefore logically trace our nursing practice we come to the root or stem from which our practice flows; these roots are identified in the principles for practice, which will be unchanging themselves, but from which our practice will grow and develop.

Accountability of the nurse

The professional nurse is accountable to her patient. To encourage each nurse to accept maximum individual responsibility and accountability, rules should be kept to a minimum, so that she can exercise her own professional judgement. Decisions about undertaking new nursing work must remain with the individual teams and their managers, and they alone should decide what new work is taken on, and what skills need to be developed.

A framework for care

With the move toward patient centred care old concepts of a sickness service are no longer appropriate. The aim of health care for each individual must be of optimal health, that is the best state of well-being possible for the patient. This entails a knowledge and understanding of the normal design and functioning of the body, exploring how disease may affect that functioning and design, and how the patient can be assisted in managing these deficiences, be they temporary, or permanent. This assistance is encapsulated in Virginia Henderson's definition of nursing.

'The unique function of the nurse is to assist the individual, sick or well in the performance of those activities contributing to health or its recovery (or to a peaceful death) that he would perform unaided if he had the necessary strength, will or knowledge.'

The patient as a person

In order to determine what assistance may be needed the nurse must consider the individual's health in terms of his functioning, including the physical, social, psychological and spiritual components. It is the balance and relationship of these various components and the response of the individual to the situation in which they find themselves, which make each person unique. Therefore, if we view patients as whole people we must consider their individual needs.

Activities of living

Human needs are complex and various, and different ones may take priority at different times. Whilst the elements of care offered to each patient will always be unique if they are to meet the needs of an individual, it is helpful to have some frame of reference to guide practice. Basic human needs are normally met by activities of daily living or self care. Nursing is concerned with meeting the deficiencies of people in carrying out daily living activities.

The process of planning nursing care

As stated earlier, a critical component in delivering nursing care is the need to develop a systematic method for making decisions about what nursing care is needed, and planning how it should be carried out. There is common recognition that certain stages must be passed through in planning nursing care. Although different nurses identify varying numbers of stages in the nursing process and give the stage different names, most of them are in effect describing the same thing: (1) assessment, (2) planning, (3) implementation, and (4) evaluation. These stages are inter-related and there is a need for re-assessment and modification of plans as evaluation takes place.

1 Assessment

The actual process of nursing requires that the nurse can make an accurate assessment of a patient's individual needs. This provides the data base for an individualized nursing plan and a baseline against which subsequent events can be compared. A nursing plan can only be as good as the information on which it is based. Assessment is not a once-only exercise, but a continuing review of the patient's condition and re-appraisal of the problems may be required. Assessment can be divided into two parts, namely, data collection and problem identification.

(a) *Data collection* is the stage at which the nurse gathers information about the patient in pre-determined categories. The primary source of information will be the patient but other sources can be used, e.g. medical records, professional colleagues, relatives, etc. Information is also gained from the nurse's observations and measurements.

(b) *Problems* are identified from the data gathered. A useful guide is to consider what is normal for the patient.

The problem may be ● actual, i.e. present at that time,

or ● potential, i.e. those that the patient is at high risk of developing.

2 Care planning

There are three major stages involved in planning care.

(a) *Setting goals*—once a problem has been identified the next stage in planning is to state briefly what kind of patient outcome the nurse, and patient, wish to achieve for each problem.

(b) *Identifying nursing intervention* which will meet the stated goals with the most appropriate nursing action, either on behalf of the patient, or assisting him to undertake his own care.

(c) *Communicating* the goals and interventions to others, which involves the use of written care plans.

3 Implementation

The stage of implementing the care plan for an individual patient means putting the plan into practice by carrying out the prescribed nursing actions. The practicalities of providing a unique programme of care for each patient need consideration. The range of dependency of the patient must be taken into account, together with the knowledge and experience of the nurse to assess and determine the need. The provision of a suitable environment and resources to give care is also a requirement. The organization and delivery of care should be undertaken by an identified nurse so that this person is accountable for the care delivered, and can ensure a consistent approach in dealing with patient problems.

4 Evaluation

Evaluation of the effectiveness of nursing care is an essential element of the nursing process. The major emphasis is placed on comparing actual patient outcomes with the stated outcome. If the care plan has stated the expected outcomes in terms of the changes the nurse expects to see in the patient over a given period of time, then it is possible to assess whether these have been achieved. This is why a clear statement of outcomes is so important. Without it evaluation of the effectiveness of nursing care becomes vague and subjective. Evaluation is a form of reassessment. Thus the dynamic nature of the nursing process is demonstrated.

Conclusion

It has been widely recognized that the nursing process is an appropriate way for nurses to bring about change in their practice in order to meet current health care needs. This 'systematic problem solving' approach to patient care is a tool which the nurse can use to steer her practice away from the traditional task-orientated approach towards a more satisfing way of meeting the total needs of the patient as an individual.

It must, however, be added that no change is easy. There is always an element of risk, since patterns of work which are familiar are easier to follow. The implementation of the Nursing Process requires much more than an alteration in the paper work; it challenges each nurse to question her practice and to have professional pride in her decision making.

Part I
Meeting Basic Needs

Maintaining Safety

International Council of Nurses Policy Statement, August 1975

'The preservation and improvement of the human environment has become a major goal of man's action for his survival and well being.'

UKCC Code of Professional Conduct, November 1984

'Each registered nurse, midwife and health visitor is accountable for his or her practice, and, in the exercise of professional accountability shall: have regard to the environment of care and its physical, psychological and social effects on patients/clients, and also to the adequacy of resources, and make known to appropriate persons or authorities any circumstances which could place patients/clients in jeopardy or which militate against safe standards of practice.'

The nurse requires a knowledge base and skills to:
- identify environmental hazards and take appropriate action,
- inform and teach preventive measures.

> ### *Normally functioning body systems*
> ### *inform the individual about his environment*

In everyday life our ability to see, hear, smell, taste and touch alert us
   to dangers, and help us to avoid them.
Memory and perceptual ability also help to ensure safety.
A person's age affects his ability to perceive, interpret and respond to
   sensory stimuli, thus additional safety precautions are needed for
   the very young or very old.
A person's emotional state affects his ability to perceive, interpret and
   respond to sensory stimuli, for example anxiety, depression,
   insecurity, or grief may increase the risk of harm from environmental hazards.

> ### *A safe, healthy environment should provide*
> ### *optimal conditions for survival, free from hazards*

Accidents may occur anywhere, at any time, but are mostly avoidable.
The nurse incorporates patient safety as her first priority in all aspects
   of patient care.
One situation which takes precedence over all others is patient safety
   in the event of fire. The nurse must know the correct action to take
   in the event of fire, and how to prevent fires occurring. Most
   hospital authorities have a mandatory requirement for staff to
   attend annual, updating, fire lectures.
Excessive noise and sensory overload may also require corrective
   action from the nurse.
Control of infection is a nursing responsibility in association with
   other members of the multidisciplinary caring team—this is
   discussed in detail in a later section.

> *Clouding or impairment of mental faculties limits the ability of the individual to interpret and respond to sensory inputs*

Sleep deprivation may distort or impair perception.

Central nervous system depressants such as alcohol and drugs dull the senses.

Illness or injury affecting the brain impair a person's ability to perceive or respond to environmental hazards.

Mental handicap or subnormality may reduce awareness of environmental dangers.

> *Impaired motor ability may reduce the opportunity for response to potentially dangerous stimuli*

The sick person may be prone to accident and injury since he may be physically weakened by his disease and impaired in his ability to care for himself.

The person in a wheelchair may be severely handicapped, he cannot move quickly and must manoeuvre the chair around objects.

A patient confined to bed, with therapeutic or diagnostic equipment in position, may be at risk and unable to protect himself.

> *Diagnostic and therapeutic measures have inherent potential for causing a patient harm*

Drug administration carries potential hazards and is discussed fully in a later section.

Radiation as a therapeutic treatment is hazardous to both patient and nurse and specific instructions *must* be followed.

Penetration of skin and invasion of body cavities renders a person vulnerable to trauma and infection—see sections on asepsis and control of infection.

Administration of local and general anaesthetics increases the risk from environmental hazards.

Guidelines for patient safety

A knowledge of safe nursing practices and preventive nursing measures is essential.

The nurse needs to be alert to any activity which could cause injury, or result in an accident.

The environment should be arranged for maximal comfort and convenience of the patient.

There should be as little clutter and as few hazardous objects in the environment as possible.

All patients have learning needs in relation to protecting themselves in a strange environment. A good orientation to the physical layout is advisable—familiarity with an environment makes it less hazardous.

The nurse should make accurate assessment of the patient's equipment needs, for example by matching heights of beds, chairs and mobility aids, particularly for the elderly or disturbed.

It is the nurse's responsibility to continuously reassess the patient's ability to protect himself from hazards, and adjust the care plan accordingly.

The nurse needs to be alert to new dangers in the environment.

All accidents or dangerous occurrences should be reported so that remedial measures can be instituted.

Communicating

Communication is complex and sophisticated.
It links people together—without it no relationship is possible.
The process of communication allows thoughts, feelings and ideas to
  be conveyed to others.

Communication is purposeful

- in order to meet physiological and safety needs,
- to form human relationships through which comfort and feelings of self esteem may be achieved,
- to exchange and compare information, for example, about illness, or needs, and the world outside the 'sickroom'.

A communication model

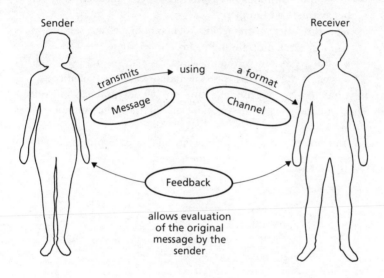

11

Communication takes two forms, non-verbal and verbal.

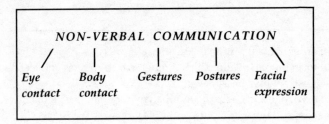

Feelings and attitudes are often conveyed through non-verbal behaviour, for example:
- posture can transmit feelings of boredom, tiredness, interest;
- gestures can indicate anger, anxiety, welcome;
- facial expression can convey love, disgust, surprise, sadness;
- eyes can be used to express incredulity, fear, lack of interest;
- touch, when appropriate, can convey thoughtfulness, empathy.

There may be cultural variations in interpretation of non-verbal behaviour.

Loss of sight, sensation, or mobility may affect both the ability to understand and to transmit messages.

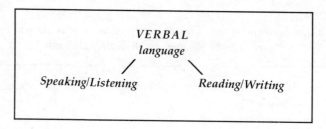

VERBAL
language

Speaking/Listening   *Reading/Writing*

The ability to read and write depends upon the stage of development of the individual, the facilities available, and the social environment.

In speaking it is not only what is said, but how it is said, that is important.

Listening is an active process in which the listener attends exclusively to the communicator.

Adjustments to the communication process may be needed in order that messages are clearly relayed and understood—for example, with the blind or deaf person.

Spoken and written communications must be understood by both the patient and the nurse.

- The language used must be the same—foreign languages, medical vocabulary and personal idiosyncrasies may affect understanding.
- Pronunciation and dialect may detract from effective communication.
- Volume, tone and speed of speech may affect the communication.
- Handwriting must be legible.
- Specialized written formats, for example, charts/computer print-out sheets, may need explanation to ensure understanding.

> *Good communication between patient and nurse is essential if care is to be planned on an individual basis*

An atmosphere should be created in which the individual feels free to communicate.

The individual's right to be different should be respected, and accepted.

Time should be allowed for communication.

Individuals involved should be aware of their own attitudes and prejudices, and not allow these to influence the communication detrimentally.

Active listening may reveal a patient's needs, problems and concerns.

The positive use of silence may comfort, and also facilitate thought and further participation in the communication process.

Fatigue may affect the special senses and reduce the capacity to receive, interpret, and transmit information effectively.

Emotions may affect the ability to communicate effectively.

Lack of motivation to enter into the interaction may render any communication ineffective.

Change in the perception of role may inhibit communication.

Knowledge of techniques which may be used to extend the communication process, for example, effective questioning, repeating key words, asking for clarification, may assist the process.

Knowledge and the use of special resources such as hearing aids, spectacles, picture boards, 'Possum' machinery, when appropriate may improve communication.

Specialists may need to be consulted, such as the speech therapist, or audiologist.

The nurse must decide:

What	——is to be communicated
Who	——is to receive the communication
Why	——she needs to communicate, and what she hopes to achieve
How	——she can best communicate the message
When	——the communication should take place
Where	——is the best place to communicate the message.

Further reading

Altschul A.T. (1980) Hints on maintaining patient-nurse interaction. *Nursing Times* **76**(15) April 10: 650–652.

Ashworth P. (1980) *Care to Communicate*. Royal College of Nursing Series, London.

Argyle M. (1972) *The Psychology of Interpersonal Behaviour*. Penguin, Harmondsworth.

Faulkner A. (1985) *Nursing—A Creative Approach*, pp 68–73. Baillière Tindall, Eastbourne.

Porritt L. (1985) *Communication—Choices for Nurses*. Churchill Livingstone, Edinburgh.

Breathing

Oxygen is essential to life—all body cells require an optimal supply in order to function efficiently.

Atmospheric air contains approximately 21% oxygen. Cellular utilization of oxygen results in the production of carbon dioxide—a waste product.

Breathing consists of movement of air into and out of the lungs in order to ensure a constant exchange of oxygen and carbon dioxide between the body and its environment, this is termed external respiration. Internal respiration is the exchange of oxygen and carbon dioxide between tissue blood capillaries and tissue cells.

> *An optimal intake of humidified and warmed oxygen is essential*

The individual needs a well ventilated environment to provide sufficient fresh air.

Supplementary oxygen, as a therapeutic substance, may be prescribed by a doctor, and administered by the nurse.

Oxygen may be administered using many different types of equipment, for example oxygen masks, nasal cannulae, and tents.

- this equipment is also prescribed, as it may influence the effectiveness of treatment.

It is important to ensure continuous flow through correct positioning and usage of oxygen equipment.

Therapeutic oxygen does not contain the natural humidity of air, so is drying to tissues.

> *A patent airway must be maintained*

The action of cilia and coughing removes mucous and foreign materials from the respiratory tract.

Positioning the patient correctly will assist in maintenance of the airway.

Obstructions to the airway must be removed, for example, dentures or vomit.

Suctioning of the upper respiratory passages may be necessary to remove secretions, if the patient is unable to cough (principles of control of infection apply).

- suctioning should not be prolonged since the patient cannot breathe adequately during this time.

Postural drainage and physiotherapy may be employed to aid removal of secretions.

Medications may be prescribed to liquefy secretions to facilitate removal.

- if this is by means of steam inhalation, care must be taken to prevent accidental scalding.

Medications may be prescribed to increase the capacity of the air passages.

> *Oxygen aids combustion and is a fire risk*

Patient safety in the presence of oxygen is paramount.

All staff should be aware of the dangers of accidental combustion.

Clear visual indication that oxygen is in use may act as an *aide-mémoire* and reduce fire risks.

Patient and visitors should be informed of the risks—explanation and continued reassurance will be necessary to gain co-operation.

Care should be taken to avoid friction and the production of sparks when oxygen therapy is in progress.

Smoking should not be allowed in the presence of oxygen, either by the patient, or anyone else in his environment.

Further reading

Chilman A. & Thomas M. (1978) *Understanding Nursing Care*. Churchill Livingstone, Edinburgh.

Evans P.M. & Massey R.M. (1979) Helping the patient with respiration. *Nursing Times* **75**(25) June 28: 1106–1107.

Levi J. (1979) Breathing equipment part 1. *Nursing* (Issue 6) September: 260–263.

Rifas E.M. (1980) How you and your patient manage dyspnoea. *Nursing Times* **80**, 10 June 6: 33–41 (includes an assessment form).

Maintaining Body Temperature

Man is classified as warm blooded or homeothermic.

Body temperature is controlled by the balance between the amount of heat produced and the amount lost.

Accurate monitoring of body temperature is an important nursing measure.

> *In health the body maintains a relatively constant temperature*
> *regardless of environmental changes,*
> *this temperature facilitates cellular activities*
> *and physiological processes*

Heat is constantly produced as a by-product of metabolism, and is gained from environmental sources.

Heat is constantly lost through evaporation, radiation, conduction, convection and excretion of body wastes, such as urine and faeces.

The base-line measurement commonly accepted for oral temperature is 37°C, but may range between 36 and 38°C.

Temperature may be measured orally, rectally, or in the axilla, using a clinical thermometer.

Other devices to record temperature include electronic thermometers, temperature monitoring probes, disposable thermometers and sensitive tape.

> *Temperature-regulating mechanisms limit the damaging effects*
> *on body tissues of extremes of heat and cold*

Temperature receptors in the skin inform the central nervous system of changes in environmental temperatures.

Impulses via the hypothalamus stimulate physiological responses to increase body temperature for example:
- muscular activity in the form of shivering,
- cellular metabolic rate increase,
- piloerection to entrap a layer of warm air next to the skin,
- cessation of sweating to limit loss of heat through evaporation of perspiration,
- surface vasoconstriction to reduce skin heat loss from conduction, convection and radiation.

Impulses via the heat-losing centre in the hypothalamus stimulate physiological responses, for example, muscular activity and metabolism decrease, and vasodilation occurs.

Behavioural responses include factors such as removal or addition of clothing, increasing or decreasing room heating or ventilation, or changing exercise patterns.

Diurnal fluctuation may occur in any one individual.

Pregnancy and ovulation cause a rise in temperature.

Menstruation causes a decrease in body temperature.

Young infants and elderly persons have less effective temperature regulating mechanisms.

Food intake affects temperature, for example, foods such as carbohydrates and fats are heat-producing substances.

Exercise increases body temperature.

A heightened emotional state increases body temperature.

In ill health body temperature fluctuation may occur in either direction outside the normal range

Fever/pyrexia

This is an elevation of the body temperature above normal.

Fever is a typical manifestation of many illnesses including: infections, diseases of the central nervous system, neoplastic and metabolic disorders.

Imbalance in body heat content may be caused by: malfunction of the temperature regulating centre, response of the centre to pyrogens, exposure to high environmental temperatures, or impaired heat dissipation.

Prolonged exposure to high environmental temperatures may induce collapse or heat stroke.

Hypothermia

This means a subnormal body temperature.

The cause may be:

- exogenous, for example, prolonged exposure to cold environmental temperatures.
- endogenous, for example, reduced metabolism, depression of body activities by alcohol intoxication, heavy sedation, or circulatory failure.

Nursing Measures

Fever/pyrexia

If the temperature is abnormally high there is a need to reduce it by
either:
- administering antipyretic drugs as prescribed by a doctor,
- surface cooling, for example fanning or tepid sponging.

Recordings of temperature and pulse should be taken at an agreed
frequency.

Skin colour and moisture state should be noted.

Rest is usually advised with temperature elevation.

Anticipation of needs may avoid unnecessary patient activity.

Information about condition and treatment may reduce anxiety and
apprehension.

Comfort measures may include:
- attention to oral hygiene,
- keeping skin clean and cool,
- change in position,
- change in bed linen and nightwear.

Nutritional state and hydration must be monitored.

Hypothermia

The immediate need is to rewarm the patient, which must be accom-
plished slowly at a rate of 5°C per hour.

Temperature should be recorded rectally for accuracy.

Measures which may be used include:
- rewarming at normal room temperature,
- use of thermal or 'space' blankets,
- immersion in a bath at an appropriate temperature,
- warmed intra-venous fluids if prescribed by a doctor.

Instability in body temperature control may persist for 7–10 days,
thus the patient should be advised to rest and be observed for this
time period.

Further reading

Du Gas B.W. (1977) *Introduction to Patient Care*, 3rd edition, Ch. 25, pp
302–478. W.B. Saunders, Philadelphia.
Watson J.E. (1979) *Surgical Nursing and Related Physiology*, 2nd edition, Ch. 6,
pp 103–110. Saunders.

Personal Hygiene

These are activities undertaken by the individual to keep his or her skin, hair, nails and mouth clean and healthy, and often form an important part of independent daily living activities.

Assisting the patient to feel well groomed may increase his or her sense of self esteem, self identity and well being.

> *Individual differences exist in the nature of the skin*
> *—changes occur in the skin throughout the life-span*

Care must be planned, on an individual basis, having taken the opportunity to listen to the patient's comments on his skin, and having assessed the state of the skin by visual and tactile means.

> *Hygiene practices vary with cultural norms,*
> *personal values and idiosyncrasies*

The nurse must familiarize herself with current practice.
In her interactions, instructions and practice the nurse must remember that these differences exist.

> *The intact skin is the body's first line of defence*
> *against infection and injury*

Skin must be washed regularly to remove harmful micro-organisms, debris, and secretions, which may damage the integrity of the skin.
Skin must be kept dry, warm, and ventilated.
An optimal diet and fluid intake is essential, and assistance may be required in the selecting and taking of a nourishing diet.
Exercise increases blood supply to the skin assisting its vitality, and the nurse must ensure that the patient has opportunity for sufficient exercise, assisting when necessary.

> *A person's general health affects the condition of his*
> *skin, nails and mucous membranes, and his ability*
> *to look after his own hygiene*

A patient may be completely independent or require assistance to maintain his own hygiene in bathroom/shower/bed or at the bedside.

Bathing should progress from the cleanest part to the least clean, from a social and microbiological viewpoint.

Attention should be paid to:
- keeping hair clean and groomed,
- nails clean and neatly cut,
- shaving, according to normal habit.

Eyes, ears and nostrils should be cleaned, if the normal cleansing mechanism is faulty. However to avoid trauma, cotton wool or instruments should not be inserted into ears, nostrils or eyes.

Oral care, when required, should include:
- cleansing of teeth and gums to remove food particles and prevent dental decay,
- cleansing of dentures and other oral appliances,
- mouthwashes to freshen the mouth and promote flow of saliva,
- application of emollients to dry or cracked lips.

Bed linen and clothing should be changed as indicated by the needs of the patient.

> *Observed changes in the skin must be reported*
> *and action initiated*

Skin and mucous membranes may be affected by:
- drugs and therapeutic treatment which may produce, for example, rashes, bruising, discoloration;
- dehydration and malnutrition, which may produce scaling, dryness, loss of elasticity or poor healing response;
- constant pressure, which may reduce blood supply to the area and may result in ischaemic ulceration.

Adverse reaction to drugs and therapeutic treatment, for example, radiotherapy, ultra-violet light, may necessitate withdrawal or modification of treatment, following consultation with medical staff.

Skin changes due to dehydration or malnutrition require reassessment of nutritional status, and adjustment to a more suitable dietary regime.

To avoid pressure it is necessary to implement a regime to reduce pressure and protect the skin:
- Change of position either for the patient, or by the patient, will relieve those areas of skin subjected to constant pressure, the frequency of change depending on the individual patient.
- Patients should be encouraged to mobilize as fully as possible.
- Correct lifting and moving should be used to prevent 'shearing' damage.
- Objects which increase pressure risk, for example, unnecessary drawsheets, waterproof sheets or crumbs in the bed should be removed.
- The correct use of aids to protect the skin such as sheepskin, bed cradles or specially designed beds should be considered.
- Skin should be kept clean, dry and as healthy as possible.

- The use of numerical scales such as the Norton scale, to identify patients at risk of developing pressure sores, may be invaluable. (This scale was designed for use in the care of the elderly. In other areas, for example acute surgery, another scale may be more appropriate.)

Physical condition		Mental condition		Activity		Mobility		Incontinence	
Good	4	Alert	4	Ambulant	4	Full	4	None	4
Fair	3	Apathetic	3	Walk/help	3	Slightly limited	3	Occasional	3
Poor	2	Confused	2	Chairbound	2	Very limited	2	Usually urine	2
Very bad	1	Stuporous	1	Bedfast	1	Immobile	1	Double	1

A score of 14 or less indicates the patient at risk.

Further reading

Blannin J.P. (1980) Towards a better life (nursing the incontinent patient). *Nursing Mirror* **150**(12) March 20: 31–33.

Harris M.D. (1980) Tools for mouth care. *Nursing Times* **74**(8) February 21: 340–342. (Data re. the acceptability of forceps, toothbrush, swab around finger were collected and analysed.)

Norton D., McLaren R. & Exton-Smith A.M. (1975) *An Investigation of Geriatric Nursing Problems in Hospital* (reprint). Churchill Livingstone, Edinburgh.

Roper N. (1976) *Man's Anatomy, Physiology, Health and Environment*, pp 125–132. Churchill Livingstone, Edinburgh.

Smith & Nephew *Pressure Sores—Pathogenesis, Prevention and Treatment*. Hill.

Eating and Drinking

A good nutritional state is reflected in, average weight for height; healthy appearance of skin, hair, eyes and mucous membranes; a good appetite; and a feeling of well being.

Food habits
- are learned, and may be beneficial or detrimental to health,
- may be related to cultural, religious or moral beliefs,
- may have psychological meaning for individuals.

> *Dietary habits may be the cause of disease*

Patterns of eating and drinking are established at an early age—education concerning diet should begin in childhood and be a life-long process.

As knowledge increases, patterns can be altered, and eating and drinking changed, to prevent or limit disease.

> *The individual requires an intake of essential nutrients and fluid, sufficient to maintain optimum health*

Assessment will help to determine normal eating and drinking patterns.

Planning of dietary intake should bear in mind nutrient and energy requirements, and the ability to take in, absorb and utilize these nutrients—thus changes will occur throughout the life span.

The individual should, whenever possible, be involved in the choice of food.

The expertise of the dietitian should be used when appropriate.

> *Nutritional status is affected by mental and physical condition*

Psychological factors such as anxiety, excitement and depression may affect eating and drinking patterns.

Physical problems such as absence of teeth, breathlessness or positional difficulties may limit the ability to eat and drink.

Systemic illness, or disease of the gastro-intestinal tract may produce anorexia, nausea, vomiting or undernourishment and change in bowel habit.

> *Disease produces a need for dietary changes
> and intake may have to be adjusted
> to suit altered body requirements*

The patient should be assisted, or supervised when necessary, with eating and drinking.

Appetite may be stimulated by:
- involving the patient in food choice,
- presenting food attractively, at the correct temperature, in appropriate form and quantity,
- an appetite stimulant, prescribed when necessary.

Undernourishment may necessitate:
- dietary supplements, such as, iron, vitamins, proteins,
- the introduction of food and fluid by artificial routes, such as:
  (i) naso-gastric tube feeding
  (ii) intravenous fluids
  (iii) total parenteral nutrition.

Measuring food and fluid intake and monitoring weight, general physical appearance and physiological status, will all provide information to evaluate care.

Some illnesses may require temporary alterations to diet and fluid intake whilst others may require a life-long change in eating and drinking habits.

Some illnesses produce nausea and vomiting—feelings of nausea may be reduced by removing from the environment anything offensive to the senses.

Anti-emetic drugs may need to be prescribed.

In the event of persistent vomiting the doctor may also prescribe naso-gastric aspiration—see guidelines.

Guidelines for naso-gastric intubation

Naso-gastric intubation may be used:

when aspiration of gastric content is required.

- the frequency of aspiration and method of drainage must be ascertained.

when naso-gastric feeding is indicated.

- the amount, frequency and type of food is prescribed.
- the feed should be given by gravity flow to prevent distension, nausea and excessive peristalsis.
- a small quantity of water instilled before and after each feed will aid the maintenance of the patency of the tube.

The patient should be positioned comfortably, in the upright position, with the neck slightly flexed to protect the air passages.

Dentures should be removed.

Clothing should be protected.

The tube is passed along the floor of the nose, down the posterior wall of the pharynx, into the oesophagus, then the stomach. Swallowing helps to ensure correct passage. Respiratory difficulty or cyanosis indicates entry of the tube into the air passages—the tube must be removed immediately.

Trauma to mucous membranes may be minimized by selection of the smallest tube compatible with the required function, and lubrication of the tube to minimize friction.

If passage of the tube induces gagging or vomiting the tube should not be advanced further until these cease. Deep breathing by the patient may minimize these effects.

Correct positioning of the tube may be ascertained by:

- aspiration of gastric content and the testing of this aspirate with litmus paper. The aspirate should be acid.
- instillation of 5 ml of air into the tube, whilst simultaneously listening with a stethoscope placed over the epigastrium. If the tube is correctly positioned air will be heard entering the stomach.

A tube remaining in position should be secured and supported to prevent dislodgement, traction, or pressure damage to the nostril.

If a tube is to be used for aspiration purposes only and no aspirate is returned, altering the position of the patient may facilitate movement of the tube within the stomach to ensure complete emptying.

A long-term naso-gastric intubation may necessitate regular changing of the tube (manufacturer's advice regarding duration of use of any particular tube should be followed). An X-ray may be required to ascertain correct position of the tube.

Withdrawal of the tube usually follows medical advice—commonly when aspirate is minimal or decreased, or when the patient is taking adequate nourishment by the oral route. On withdrawal the tube should be clamped to avoid fluid entering the respiratory tract.

Requirements for naso-gastric intubation

Naso-gastric tube of appropriate size and length
Receiver and tissues
Syringe
Litmus paper and stethoscope
Spigot, drainage bag and feeding equipment
Adhesive tape
Receptacle for used materials
Mouthwash on completion of the insertion for patient comfort.

Guidelines for care—central venous catheterization for parenteral feeding or measurement purposes

NB *The placement of a cannula into a central vein is always a medical responsibility and is potentially hazardous, with infection and air embolus risks.* **Only qualified nurses who have received appropriate training should take responsibility for parenteral feeding and care of the cannula.**

In all cases of parenteral feeding the expertise of the nutrition nurse should be sought.

For subclavian cannulation the patient assumes the supine position with a pillow placed longitudinally down the back to encourage the shoulders to fall back, thus raising the clavicle and facilitating puncture of the vein.

Following insertion, radiological confirmation of the cannula position should be obtained.

Pain, dyspnoea or cyanosis should be reported to medical staff immediately since they may indicate pneumothorax, a potential complication.

The infusion should run continuously to prevent blockage of the catheter. Alternatively, the installation of heparinized saline may be prescribed. Care must be taken to ensure the equipment does not disconnect.

Skin around the entry site is cleaned regularly using a strict aseptic technique and an approved antiseptic solution. The entry site is covered with a sterile, occlusive dressing, which must also prevent movement of the cannula.

For removal, the patient assumes the supine position to prevent air embolism occurring, and a small occlusive dressing is placed over the exit site.

The nurse checks that the catheter is complete and the tip is sent to the laboratory for culture and sensitivity.

Requirements

In addition to the requirements for routine intravenous cannulation the following should be provided:

Local anaesthetic, syringes, needles

Sterile gowns, gloves and large drapes

The required cannula

Skin cleansing agents—the established antiseptic detailed by hospital policy, with the addition of povidone iodine
Suturing materials
Adhesive tape.

Further reading

Amos A. (1976) Parenteral nutrition—the nurse's role. *Nursing Times* **72**(30) July 29: 1153–1155.
Bateman J.M. (1979) Helping the patient with eating and drinking. *Nursing Times* **75**(23) June 7: 957–959.
Coates V. (1985) *Are they being served?* Royal College of Nursing.
Du Gas B.W. (1983) *Introduction to Patient Care*, 4th edition, Ch. 14, pp 259–302. Saunders International, Philadelphia.
Jenner A.E. (1977) Intravenous infusion—a cause for concern? *Nursing Times* **73**(5) February 3: 156–158.

Eliminating

Elimination of metabolic waste products is essential to efficient body function.

Routes of elimination include micturition, defaecation, expiration and perspiration.

Interruption of the normal excretory mechanisms produces serious consequences for body functioning since waste products may be retained, and body fluid and electrolyte balance disordered.

> *Independent control of urinary and faecal elimination*
> *is gained in childhood*

A loss of dignity and self esteem may occur if problems with urinary and faecal elimination require medical or nursing intervention.

Medical and nursing intervention may produce embarrassment for both patient and staff.

> *Individuals develop their own elimination habits and patterns*

There may be social and cultural differences in elimination habits and patterns.

Assessment will ensure care planning creates optimal conditions for elimination for each patient.

Accurate recording of output, and evaluation of care, will aid continuity and future planning.

> *Physical factors may affect elimination*

The quantity and quality of diet and fluid intake may increase, or decrease elimination.

Immobility may produce physiological effects on elimination as well as problems in the use of equipment and facilities.

Systemic illness and disorders of the urinary and gastro-intestinal tract may produce alterations in elimination.

As a secondary effect, certain drugs stimulate or suppress elimination.

Medications may be specifically prescribed to stimulate or suppress elimination.

Fear and anxiety may alter the patient's normal pattern of elimination.

Loss of privacy and embarrassment may restrict the ability to eliminate.

Language used to describe elimination must be determined at assessment, by both patient and nurse, to avoid misunderstanding.

Information, discussion of problems and prompt attention may help to reduce the psychological stresses for the patient.

Environmental factors may affect elimination

Facilities must be available for all patients:
- the bathroom or toilet is the ideal place for elimination—aids, such as handrails, and raised toilet seats may assist the patient in retaining independence.
- when required, equipment such as commodes, bedpans or urinals must be handled competently and correctly. (The principles of control of infection apply.)

The area used for elimination purposes must be warm and ventilated—unnecessary exposure of the patient must be avoided.

Time must be allowed to suit individual needs.

Privacy must be ensured, whenever possible,
- if total privacy is ensured, the patient must feel secure in the knowledge that nursing help is available as soon as required.

Facilities for personal hygiene must be available after elimination.

> *Nursing intervention may be required to assist elimination*

Urinary elimination:

A monitored or increased fluid intake may be necessary.

The most convenient and comfortable position for voiding should be adopted.

The application of warmth to the lower abdomen and perineal area may relax tense muscles.

If prescribed by the doctor, urethral catheter insertion may be necessary.

Faecal elimination:

Can be affected by adjustments in dietary intake.

A comfortable position should be adopted.

Alterations to mobility patterns may be required to assist more normal bowel functioning, since exercise helps to stimulate gut movement.

Medications prescribed orally or rectally may increase or diminish elimination.

Rectal medications may be given in the form of enemas or suppositories.

Some people have altered excretory routes, for example patients with a:
- colostomy,
- ileal conduit.

The formation of an artificial opening for discharging of excreta may produce fear, anxiety and/or change in perceived body image.

Severe urinary and faecal elimination problems may require urgent medical intervention, for example:
- renal failure requiring haemodialysis,
- acute intestinal obstruction requiring surgery.

Guidelines for urethral catheterization and drainage

The principles of asepsis and control of infection apply.

The risk of trauma is reduced by using a catheter of appropriate size and type to meet the patient's needs.

To prevent trauma and friction a sterile lubricant may be used for insertion.

To reduce trauma and irritation catheter and tubing should be supported.

To ensure unobstructed outflow the system should be prevented from kinking, and the drainage bag kept below the level of the bladder. However, at no time must any part of the equipment rest on the floor.

The bag should be emptied regularly to avoid overfilling, which can lead to drag on the catheter.

If an indwelling catheter has been inserted then a closed drainage system must be maintained. Unnecessary changing of the drainage bag increases infection risk. A bag should only be changed if there is leakage, or if the urine is offensive or infected.

If continuity of the closed drainage system is interrupted the catheter outlet should be thoroughly cleansed with a bactericidal solution, and a new, sterile drainage bag connected.

To reduce infection risk the genital area must be kept clean by regular washing.

In specialized areas an aseptic catheter toilet, using a solution such as normal saline may be employed at regular intervals.

Alternative methods of bladder drainage, which carry fewer risks, should always be considered, e.g. penile sheath or manual compression of bladder.

Requirements:

CSSD catheterization pack
Appropriate selection of catheters
Sterile disposable gloves
Cleansing lotions
Lubricating solutions
Sterile water to inflate catheter balloon
Drainage bag and holder
Scissors and adhesive tape
Measuring jug
Specimen bottles
Receptacles for used materials and instruments.

Guidelines for administration of enemas, suppositories and rectal washout

NB *Medicated enemas and suppositories are prescribed—the principles of drug administration apply.*

If possible the patient assumes the left lateral position with the right leg acutely flexed—thus the sigmoid colon lies below the level of the rectum.

Relaxation of the anal sphincter may be promoted if the patient breathes deeply.

Friction and trauma to mucous membranes will be reduced by using a lubricant.

Fluids administered rectally should be at body temperature.

Inserting fluid under pressure rectally may induce contraction of the intestinal wall, and pain, and should therefore be avoided.

Raising the foot of the bed, and ensuring bladder and bowel are empty prior to administration, may help when retention enemas or suppositories are prescribed.

Evacuant suppositories should be retained for some time prior to evacuation—evacuant enemas are returned immediately.

For rectal washout in an adult, not more than 300 ml of fluid should be inserted at any one time, prior to siphoning back.

Requirements

Protection for the bed
Prescribed enemas and suppositories
Disposable gloves
Lubricant

Toilet facilities should have been prepared.

Hygiene facilities should be available for the patient on completion.

Guidelines for stoma care

Pre-operatively

The site of the stoma should be identified, preferably by a stoma care nurse, to accommodate such factors as skin creases and folds, old scars, belt line, avoiding rib cage, groin and pelvic bones; patients are asked to adopt different positions to assess the ideal stoma site.

The patient may be tested for allergies to adhesives, plastic, etc. all of which may be used in the manufacture of stoma appliances, although with modern appliances this is now less of a problem.

There is a vast range of stoma equipment available and it is usual to limit the initial information on appliances to the post-operative bags and flanges—but if the patient asks to see more, information should be forthcoming.

In the pre-operative phase it is vital to note the physical condition of the patient, e.g. poor eyesight, arthritis in the hands, or the presence of congenital deformities. Perhaps more importantly the psychological reaction must be noted. It may be relief at the end of the symptoms of disease such as ulcerative colitis, or total disquiet or fear due to underlying disease of unknown aetiology. Many need a great deal of pre-operative counselling, which should be given by the stoma care nurse in co-operation with nursing and medical staff.

Post-operatively

Observations include:

looking at the colour of the stoma, which should be red—any colour changes, e.g. dusky, blue or black should be reported to medical staff immediately.

The post-operative appliance should be a two piece design, with clean drainable bag.

The peristomal skin is best protected by a stomahesive or similar wafer with flange incorporated. Any signs of soreness are reported.

The stoma size should be measured accurately and an appliance of the correct size fitted (noting that newly formed stomas tend to be oedematous and do shrink.) Too large a flange will leave skin exposed and allow effluent to make peristomal skin sore, too small a flange will aid occlusion of the blood supply and lead to ischaemia, necrosis and stenosis.

On each bag change the peristomal skin and stoma should be carefully inspected. Skin cleansing is done with warm water and tissues or soap if required, avoiding the use of other cleansing agents and solvents. The skin must be dried thoroughly before fitting a fresh appliance.

Regular assessment should be made of the nature and amount of output from the stoma—excessive watery loss should be reported to medical staff immediately—this is especially relevant with new ileostomists since dehydration may quickly ensue.

The drainage bag should be emptied when half full noting the presence of flatus as well as effluent.

The effectiveness of the appliance should be regularly evaluated; a leaking appliance should never be patched but replaced with an appliance of the correct size immediately.

Dietary changes

May be necessary until the patient adjusts to the altered excretory pathway.

Colostomists and ileostomists

Foods often blamed for producing excessive odour and flatus include beans, eggs, cabbage, fish and onions.

Initially carbonated drinks and beer may also have to be avoided.

A modern plastic appliance with flatus filter or drainable clamp should dispel odours.

In the early post-operative phase an ostomy deodorant, e.g. Nilodor or Ozium, may be necessary or a charcoal tablet in the bag.

Ileostomists

May need to add salt and extra fluid to the diet if there is a high output from the stoma.

Urinary diversion patients

(Urostomy and ileal loop conduit stoma)

May need to increase fluid intake and be taught how to identify urinary tract infections. The urine will contain mucous if an ileal conduit is formed—this is different from the cloudiness and smell associated with infection.

NB *Unless there is a risk of cross infection, gloves should never be worn when attending to a stoma.*

> *It is important to seek specialist guidance if any
> stoma problems arise. If the nurse fails to deal
> expertly with the problems this will only confirm the
> patient's view that this is difficult to deal with.
> Any mistakes made, for example not fitting
> the appliance correctly, leading perhaps to leakage,
> will also lower the patient's morale and may
> inhibit recovery*

Further reading

Breckman B.E. (1977) Care of the stoma patient. *Nursing Mirror Supplement* **145**(15) October 13: i–iv.

Browne B. (1979) *Management for Continence*. Age Concern Booklet, London.

Gumbrell J. (1976) The ileal conduit patient. *Nursing Mirror* **143**(a) August 26: 54–55.

Lewin D. (1976) Care of the constipated patient. *Nursing Mirror* **72**(12) March 25: 444–446.

Meers P.D. & Stronge J.L. (1980) Hospitals should do the sick no harm (7). Urinary tract infections. *Nursing Times* **76**(30) July 24.

Smart M. & Ali N. (1980) Long-term catheters—questions nurses ask. *Nursing Times Community Outlook* **76**(15) April 10: 107–110.

Mobilizing

All living creatures move.

Movement contributes to the enjoyment of life, and is essential in the maintenance of homeostasis, enabling the body to respond to changes in both its external and internal environments.

Moving forms an essential part of the behaviours required in everyday living.

> **An individual with limited mobility needs to maintain
> and regain maximal independence**

Assessment of the patient's mobility is crucial to planning appropriate
help.
  - some patients may be largely dependent; for example, people
    who are quadriplegic.
  - some patients may be semi-dependent; for example, those with
    fractured limbs.
  - some patients may have restricted movement due to pain or
    deformity; for example, people with arthritis.
  - some patients may be independent, needing advice only.
Purposeful movement, ambulation and exercise depend upon the
    stage of physical development of an individual.
Information is required about the nature and extent of deviation from
    the norm, and the patient's adaptation to limitations, so that he
    may perform his activities of daily living.
Mechanical devices which can be used by the patient for independent
    movement should be readily available and conveniently situated
    to obviate his having to ask for unnecessary assistance.
The expertise of the physiotherapist and occupational therapist are
    invaluable for maintaining maximal patient independence.

> **When mobility is impaired the patient may need help
> to perform the activities of daily living**

Breathing may be difficult if mobility is restricted.
Hygiene practices may require adjustment.
Dietary intake may need to be altered.
Limited mobility may produce changes in bowel and bladder
    function. Assistance may be required with the use of facilities for
    elimination.
Inability to move normally may cause anger, distress, frustration or
    inappropriate dependence. This will require appropriate infor-
    mation giving, instruction, psychological support and encourage-
    ment.

> *When help is required in moving, the imposed load on the assistant(s) can result in physical overstress*

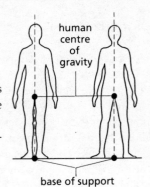

human centre of gravity

base of support

Stability of the assistant is greater when there is a wide base of support.

The base will be wider and therefore safer if the feet are apart.

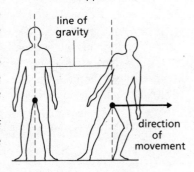

line of gravity

direction of movement

Stability is maintained if the line of gravity falls within the base of support.

When moving the patient the assistant(s) should keep the body in alignment over the wide base of support.

This is achieved by a series of short lifts re-aligning the body between each lift.

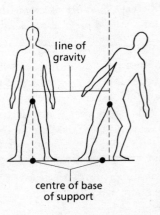

line of gravity

centre of base of support

Less energy is required to maintain balance when the line of gravity falls nearest the centre of the base of support.

If a stooping posture is maintained for a time this can cause muscle strain.

> *Energy must be used efficiently when assisting the patient*

The amount of energy required to move an object depends upon the resistance of the object as well as the gravitational pull.

The friction between an object and the surface on which it is moved affects the amount of energy needed to complete the movement.

Less energy is required to push, pull or slide an object than to lift it—if this technique is used for a patient, then care must be taken to avoid trauma by friction.

Less energy is required if the weight of the assistant is used to counter-balance the patient's weight.

Less energy is expended if equipment such as a hoist is used to lift or move a patient. Never lift manually unless you really have to.

Green's mobility assessment scale

A score of 10 or more indicates that *one person alone cannot help* the patient to move without risking injury to either patient or assistant.

Weight	Physical disability	Co-operation	Level of consciousness	Muscular strength
Up to 6 kg 1 (≈ 1 stone)	Restricted 1 use of one limb	Good 1	Alert 1	Normal 1
6–19 kg 2 (≈ 1–3 stone)	Restricted 2 use of two limbs	Fair 2	Drowsy 2	Fair 2
19–25 kg 3 (≈ 3–4 stone)	Restricted 3 use of three limbs	Poor 3	Semi-conscious 3	Weak 3
Over 25 kg 4 (Over 4 stone)	Restricted 4 use of four limbs	Uncooperative 4	Unconscious 4	Very weak 4

In order to complete lifting or moving of any patients successfully, make time to assess the load and the environment and think before you act.

Prepare the patient
- explain what you intend to do,
- consult, to confirm the patient's preferences,
- obtain his assistance and co-operation,
- adjust extraneous equipment as required, such as catheters or drainage equipment.

Prepare the assistants
- have sufficient assistance to complete the lift or move safely,
- decide the appropriate action and appoint a leader,
- instruct each assistant in his/her role.
- remove personal objects which may injure the patient such as fob watches or name badges.

Prepare the environment and equipment
- clear the area of unnecessary objects,
- obtain necessary aids,
- adjust heights where possible,
- apply brakes to mobile equipment.

Apply basic rules
- stand with feet apart,
- bend hips and knees,
- brace back to keep straight,
- hold object close, using a firm grip,
- lift by standing up,
- bend knees to lower patient.

> *Assessment of the patient will determine whether help is required to lift or move him—IF IN DOUBT NEVER LIFT OR MOVE A PATIENT UNAIDED*

Further reading

Chilman A. & Thomas M. (1978) *Understanding Nursing Care*, pp 29–40. Churchill Livingstone, Edinburgh.

Hollis M. (1985) *Safer Lifting for Patient Care*, 2nd edition. Blackwell Scientific Publications, Oxford.

Johnston M. (1985) *Assessment and Planning prior to Patient Mobilization*. Unpublished research project by a Clinical Teacher. Copy held at Regional Offices, Oxfordshire Health Authority.

Lloyd P. (1981) *The Handling of Patients—a guide for nurse managers*. Royal College of Nursing in conjunction with the Back Pain Association.

Recreation—Rest/Relaxation, Sleeping

Each person establishes his own pattern of work, recreation, rest, relaxation, and sleep. This pattern affords the individual the greatest physical and emotional satisfaction and helps to maintain health.

Recreation implies pleasurable occupation—it invigorates the individual.

Rest and relaxation, imply repose, a lessening of tension, refreshing inactivity and freedom from disturbance.

Sleep is a period of rest for body and mind, involving relaxation of consciousness and a lessening of physical activity, allowing body cells a time for growth and repair.

> *The purpose of recreation is the enjoyment of leisure time and the prevention of boredom and discontentment*

Recreational activities should be:
- interesting and varied,
- involve different activities from those imposed by daily living,
- a change of activity, stimulating conversation, or simply a change of environment may be recreational—recreation does not necessarily require physical activity,
- facilities may include the media, games rooms, library and occupational therapy services.

> *Recreation should be compatible with, and conducive to, physical, mental and social well being*

Relatives and visitors may wish to be included in the recreational activities of the patient.
Provision for recreation should take into consideration:
- age, physical and psychological ability,
- cultural and religious beliefs,
- environmental and economic constraints,
- motivation and requirement.

> *Illness may interfere with recreational abilities*

The acutely ill patient concentrates energy on 'getting well' and may not be interested in recreation.
Long term illness may prevent the individual from pursuing his preferred activities—this may produce frustration or anger.

> *Optimal rest, relaxation, and sleep is only possible if*
> *the individual is free from physical and psychological discomfort*

Physical discomfort includes such things as pain, inappropriate environmental temperature, hunger or thirst, and excessive noise or light.

Psychologial discomfort includes feelings such as fear, loneliness, excitement, depression and anxiety.

The use of a variety of relaxation techniques such as hypnosis , yoga or massage may promote rest and sleep.

> *Every individual has his own sleep rhythm*
> *and therefore individual sleep requirements*

Sleep patterns are influenced by a person's age, physical and mental state, social and environmental conditions.

Sleep occurs in cycles, 4–6 cycles are thought to occur during a normal sleep period, each cycle having several stages:

- drowsiness—a slowing down of activity, the person may be wakened with slight stimulus;
- greater relaxation—after about 15 minutes, easily awakened;
- complete relaxation—after about 30 minutes, may move or speak;
- deep sleep—difficult to awaken, bed wetting or sleep walking may occur in some individuals during this stage;
- light sleep—REM (rapid eye movement) sleep, dreaming occurs.

> *Sleep deprivation may have a profound effect*
> *on physical and mental functioning*

- irritability and anxiety are likely to increase;
- concentration and memory may be impaired;
- the individual may feel lethargic and depressed;
- resistance to infection is lowered and tissue repair diminished.

> *Illness and hospitalization are likely to produce sleep deprivation*

Factors which affect sleep rhythms include:
Environmental
- sharing a room with others,
- change in bed or bed linen.

Physical
- problems in achieving a comfortable position,
- a full bladder, pain or nausea,
- the need to be awakened for therapeutic or monitoring purposes.

Psychological
- anxiety regarding treatment or prognosis.

NB *Observation, foresight and knowledge may prevent or alleviate problems.*

Possible nursing and medical interventions include:
- provision of a daily routine which follows the patient's normal pattern,
- provision of diversional activities during waking hours,
- administration of prescribed medication.

Further reading

Esson E. (1970) Nurse, could you care more? *Nursing Times* **75**(33) August 16: 1387–1388. (Useful information about nursing on night duty to ensure patients sleep well.)

Oswald I. (1974) *Sleep.* Penguin, Harmondsworth.

Martin I.C.A. (1978) Aspects of relaxation technique. *Nursing Times* **74**(23) June 8: 953–955.

Expressing Sexuality

The sexual drive, or libido, is a basic physiological need, a powerful motivating force essential to survival of the species.

Complex psycho-social relationships accompany the expression of sexual need.

> *With few exceptions, the male and female sexual identity*
> *is determined at conception*

An important developmental task after birth is the formation of gender identity, and the ability to express the quality of being male/female.

Sexual identity is often bound up in the social role adopted, even in the 'western' culture where traditional roles are becoming blurred.

The ability to express sexual identity may be important in gaining recognition from others and love and companionship.

The ability to express sexuality may depend on the person's self perception and self esteem. These may depend on personal appearance as well as the role the person adopts.

Clothing and behaviour may be adjusted to portray the required sexual identity.

> *Physiological factors may affect*
> *the expression of sexuality in health*

Endocrine production of the sex hormones must be within normal limits.

Age and stage of physical development affect the sexual drive.

- Adolescence produces maturation of the sexual organs, the differentiation of the male/female form, and may induce increased interest in sexual activity.
- Women have a finite reproductive timespan although the sexual drive is not necessarily limited by this.
- Men continue to produce spermatozoa into old age and therefore remain capable of reproduction.
- Ageing, when atrophy of the reproductive system occurs, may reduce sexual function.

Disability may affect functioning: for example, impotence following pelvic floor surgery.

> ## *Psychological factors may affect the expression of sexuality*

Loss of privacy and dignity may induce embarrassment about sexuality.

Lack of information regarding the sexual act may affect sexual capability.

Anxiety or fear: for example, of unwanted pregnancy, or contracting sexually transmitted disease may limit activity.

Repressed childhood emotions and psychological damage caused by early childhood experiences may affect expression of sexuality.

Ageing may produce worries about sexual attractiveness or potency.

> ## *Social, cultural and religious factors may affect expression of sexuality*

Each culture exerts its own controls on acceptable sexual behaviour.

Social attitudes towards the type of sexual relationship encountered may have an effect: for example, incest whilst unacceptable in the United Kingdom, may be acceptable in certain other cultures.

Sexual taboos may be emphasized by legal sanctions, some sexual acts being considered criminal: for example, rape and child molesting are criminal acts in the United Kingdom.

The religious beliefs held may affect expression of sexuality.

Long term institutionalization: for example, in prison, or hospitalization may limit opportunities for expressing sexuality.

Disorder of the reproductive system such as tumour, or infection, may affect sexual functioning.

Systemic disorders, such as cardiovascular disease, or the malaise of chronic illness, may limit sexual activity.

Conditions affecting mobility and co-ordination: for example, multiple sclerosis, parkinsonism or 'stroke', may affect sexual activity.

Drugs or surgical treatments may disrupt sexual functioning, as may interventions such as catheterization of the bladder.

Disruption of self-image: for example, hair loss following cytotoxic therapy, or facial surgery, may affect the expression of sexuality.

Nursing actions include:

Acceptance of sexuality needs in the patient even if these do not comply with those held personally.

A calm, professional manner in dealing with giving sexual information, which should be adequate for the needs of the patient, and may alter as the health status of the patient alters.

Careful assessment of need, for example:
- the patient may request only a nurse or doctor of the same sex present during investigations or treatments;
- a member of the older generation may not wish to discuss personal matters except with the doctor.

The provision of privacy and maintenance of patient dignity during assessment, and when carrying out planned care.

Ensuring minimum disruption of existing close relationships.

Eliciting expert help where necessary: for example, a psychotherapist, sexual counsellor, member of Mastectomy Association.

Further reading

Du Gas B.W. (1983) *Introduction to Patient Care*, 4th edition, Ch. 29, pp 635–659. Saunders International, Philadelphia.

Spiritual Comfort

The concept of spiritual belief varies from person to person.

Spiritual belief reflects an awareness, on the part of the individual, of an inner strength, which sustains and motivates him.

Religion is, for many people, an important element in their lives. Others realize their spiritual needs outside a formal religion.

> *A religious belief, ethical concepts, moral values, and*
> *motivating forces lie at the centre of most individuals' lives*

Each person is unique, and develops a particular combination of
beliefs, hopes, fears and values, derived from what has been
taught, learned from experience, and by intuition.

The achievement of health is to some extent dependent on harmony
between belief and behaviour.

Illness, which may produce changes in lifestyle or the possibility of
death, may shake the individual's belief or create new spiritual
needs.

> *There are many varieties of spiritual philosophy, any of*
> *which may help a person to attain or maintain peace of mind*

A relationship must be established between the patient and nurse,
which facilitates the expression of spiritual needs and practices.

Tolerance and respect should be shown towards the spiritual philosophies of others.

Facilities should be available to enable the patient to live or die within
the tenets of his faith.

For example:
- recognition of hygiene practices,
- alternatives to prohibited foods,
- recognition of religious celebrations and holidays,
- observance of accepted practices following death.

The hospital chaplain is part of the caring team, and his help and
advice should be sought when appropriate.

The patient's own minister of religion and friends or relatives who
share the patient's belief should be welcomed. They may be
involved in caring for the patient and his spiritual needs. Their
experience, expertise and advice may be essential.

Some patients may hold no religious beliefs. In these circumstances it
is inappropriate that the nurse imposes her own beliefs.

> *Certain spiritual philosophies may have a direct bearing*
> *on the patient's illness and recovery*

Alternative or complementary medicine employs such theories as faith healing, meditation or prayer, as part of management and treatment.

Some philosophies may require the patient to refuse specific therapies,

> e.g. Jehovah's Witnesses may refuse blood transfusion.
>> Christian Scientists may refuse drug treatments.

These beliefs may need to be incorporated in the patient's care plan.

Further reading

Richards F. (1978) What they are and what they believe. *Nursing Mirror*.
Part 1. Roman Catholics, Jehovah Witnesses, Christian Scientists. **144**(15) April 14: 65–66.
Part 2. The Jewish Faith. April 21: 64.
Part 3. Muslims, Hindus, Buddhists. April 28: 67, 80.

Terminal Illness and Death

The underlying aim of terminal care is to help people to die, in comfort, and with dignity, whilst retaining individuality. An atmosphere must be created in which adjustment to death can be encouraged and helped. Death should be seen as an acceptable part of life.

To meet the emotional needs of the dying the carer must understand the psychological stages that people approaching death encounter.

Non-acceptance/denial	—'there must be some mistake'
Anger/hostility	—'why me?'—criticism of carers or God
Bargaining	—promise of good behaviour to bring about reversal of imminent death, or relief of pain
Depression	—putting affairs in order—withdrawal
Acceptance	—feelings of peace

> *The central focus of good terminal care*
> *is the recognition of the individuality*
> *of the person who is dying*

Caring involves the development of relationships:

- it is important that the nurse knows the degree of knowledge each patient has of his inevitable death, as this may affect the relationship.
- the patient should be allowed to express feelings and emotions about his approaching death in his own way.

Individualized patient care should replace inflexible routines.

Skilled treatment of physical symptoms will allow the patient to remain comfortable, and, as much as possible, in control of the remainder of his life.

Individuality is enhanced by the patient wearing his own clothes—the presence of treasured personal possessions may give great psychological comfort.

> *A relaxed atmosphere generates feelings of peace*
> *and comfort for the terminally ill*

Distress may be caused by care which is hurried and perfunctory—a calm, relaxed nurse, willing to spend time with the patient, may more easily inspire trust and confidence.

Unnecessary noise and activity should be avoided in order to ensure optimal conditions for sleep and rest.

Open visiting ensures friends and relatives are present whenever needed, and avoids the tension and noise of set visiting hours.

Comfort may be gained from allowing children or pets to visit.

The patient should feel free to arrange his environment and his day to suit himself, and to participate in his own care whenever he has the necessary strength and will—this may increase his self-esteem and self-identity.

The patient's environment should be neat and tidy—visual beauty in the surroundings is often important to the dying.

> *Care is aimed at alleviating physical and*
> *psychological symptoms, to allow the*
> *person to live his remaining life to the full*

The control of physical pain and psychological symptoms must be regularly evaluated to ensure that treatment is effective.

Breathlessness may be eased by correct positioning, environmental ventilation, reassurance, and therapeutic oxygen if prescribed.

Constipation, which may occur as a result of medication, under-nourishment, lack of exercise or poor fluid intake, should be alleviated.

Personal hygiene is adjusted to the needs of the patient and may include the management of incontinence and the prevention of pressure sore development.

Feelings of isolation and loneliness can be prevented by ensuring physical and social contact.

Effective communication between the patient, his family and the nurse should ensure that they are prepared for any crisis.

Many patients find their religious beliefs of great help in preparing to face death—the assistance of the minister of religion should be sought if requested by the patient.

Hearing is thought to be one of the last senses to diminish and communication should be maintained even if the patient cannot respond.

Relatives/friends should be regarded as key members of the caring team, and the presence of a trusted friend or relative may afford the patient great comfort and reassurance.

The nurse should give support and guidance to the relatives, who may feel less helpless if they are allowed to participate actively in care.

Skilled counselling support may be required to help relatives deal with their feelings regarding illness and death.

Accommodation, catering facilities, and financial assistance may be required and the social worker may need to assist.

Grieving relatives or friends should never be hurried away.

Facilities should be made available for private expression of grief and religious beliefs.

The body and the environment should be carefully prepared to reduce distress when relatives visit.

After death the patient's spiritual philosophy may influence physical care.

After last offices are completed, the body may be moved to an appropriate environment, such as a Chapel of Rest.

Requests made by the patient before death, such as organ donation, should be honoured.

> *When a person dies there are legal issues which require attention*

The identity of the body must be ensured.

Personal possessions and valuables are made ready for the relatives.

Relatives may be offered advice regarding registration of death and funeral arrangements.

Post mortem examination may be requested by the doctor—under certain circumstances this is a legal requirement.

The death certificate must be signed by the doctor.

Guidelines for last offices

Religious beliefs should have been ascertained, and respected.

Relatives may express a wish to be involved in the process and this request must be facilitated.

The body should be placed flat, with limbs straight, eyes and mouth closed—prostheses, such as dentures should be replaced.

Certain religious beliefs require a time lapse before further intervention (one hour is usually accepted practice).

Any equipment used for treatment, such as naso-gastric, rectal, urinary and intravenous catheters may be removed.

Wound drainage tubes may be cut short and left in position, sealed to prevent leakage.

Wounds should be redressed and sealed.

Pacemaker wires should be left in position and note made of this.

NB *Some items of equipment may be required to be left in position in the case of post mortem requests.*

The bladder should be emptied by manual compression if this has not happened reflexly.

Washing, shaving, and grooming of the hair may be performed.

The patient's clothing is replaced by a shroud.

Jewellery is removed, unless otherwise indicated by the patient or relatives—if left in place this must be recorded.

The patient's identity label is left in position.

The body is wrapped and secured in a mortuary sheet.

Identification labels are attached to the body and the mortuary sheet.

Possessions and valuables are checked and listed carefully and safe custody is ensured until the next of kin can take possession.

The body is removed from the ward area to the mortuary.

Post mortem requests, and death notices, are completed by the appropriate member of staff and forwarded to the correct departments.

Further reading

Brown E.A. (1979) Personal experience on the care of the dying. *Nursing Times* **75**(13) March 29: 545–546.

Charles-Edwards A. (1983) *The Nursing Care of the Dying Patient.* Beaconsfield Publishing Ltd, Beaconsfield.

Kubler-Ross E. (1970) *On Death and Dying.* Tavistock Publications, London.

Penson J.M. (1979) Helping the bereaved. *Nursing Times* **75**(14) April 5: 593–595.

Stedeford A. (1978) *Facing Death.* Heinemann, London.

Part II
Other Components of Care

Drug Administration

Therapeutic drugs are powerful agents used in the prevention and treatment of disease, and in the alleviation or control of symptoms of ill health.

Modern drugs are powerful in their effects for good or for harm; appropriate use, knowledge about their effects, and accurate administration is essential for the effective care of patients. Ignorant or careless administration of drugs can be dangerous to patients, and may reduce their effectiveness.

The type of drug, and/or the patient's health problems may determine the route of administration

---

Drugs may be administered—
Orally
- this is relatively convenient, economic and comfortable for the patient, who must possess swallowing abilities and absorption potential from the gastro-intestinal tract,
- sublingual drugs may be ineffective if swallowed.

By injection
- the principles of asepsis and control of infection apply;
- injection sites must be free from lesions or scar tissue;
- injection sites should be alternated for patients requiring repeated injections.

subcutaneous injections
- allow small amounts of a drug to be introduced into the soft tissues just beneath the skin.

intramuscular injections
- allow larger quantities of fluid/drug to be administered, and decreases absorption time.

intravenous injection
- used when rapid drug effects are required or constant blood serum of a drug is needed, or when large fluid quantities are required to dilute a drug;
- only medical staff and qualified nurses who are trained and assessed as competent in the use of this route may give intra-venous injections.

By inhalation
- the drug is absorbed into the blood vessels of the upper respiratory tract for direct, or distant systemic effect.

Topically
- the drug is applied to, and absorbed through, the skin.

By instillation
- the drug is instilled into body cavities, for example, nose, ears or rectum, and absorbed through the mucosa into the blood stream.

> *Nurses may not prescribe drugs in normal circumstances*

Drug prescription is the legal responsibility of the doctor. This responsibility cannot be delegated—outcomes from the prescription, for example, side effects and incompatibilities, remain the responsibility of the doctor.

> **The nurse has a professional duty to carry out the medical prescription accurately, and to ensure that the patient comes to no harm from any act or omission on her part**

To facilitate safe administration, the nurse requires considerable knowledge and skill:

- Knowledge of the patient, and the role of drug therapy in the planning of care.
- Knowledge of local policies and statutory drug rules regarding safe custody, storage, and administration.
- Knowledge of classes of drugs and their:
    therapeutic action,
    side effects,
    drug incompatabilities,
    dosages,
    administration routes.
- Ability to interpret prescription sheets and:
    calculate drug dosages,
    administer drugs safely and accurately by prescribed routes,
    maintain accurate records.

> **Care must be taken when handling drugs, since local or systemic idiosyncratic reactions may occur following exposure**

When administering drugs the nurse must administer

the	*right medication*	Identify
	in	
the	*right dosage*	Check
	to	
the	*right patient*	Verify
	by	
the	*right route*	Recheck
	at	
the	*right time*	Record

***The therapeutic value of any drug may be enhanced
or decreased by the way it is stored or administered***

Certain drugs are administered in specific formats and note should be taken of this when considering administration, for example:
- enteric coated tablets must not be crushed,
- liquid oral preparations may need to be shaken to distribute the drug evenly.

After taking any drug orally, a small amount of liquid should be given to ensure irritation of the oesophagus is reduced to a minimum, and rapid transmission to the stomach occurs.

The timing of drug administration may be crucial to the effect and should therefore be adhered to, for example, before or with food, or during the night, which may necessitate waking the patient.

Nursing care measures may help to enhance drug action, such as correct positioning of the patient for inhaled or instilled drugs.

To minimize transmission of micro-organisms or absorption of the drug, the nurse should avoid handling a drug and wash and dry hands before, and when necessary, during, drug administration.

Drugs should be kept at optimum temperatures to avoid deterioration.

Drugs shold not be exposed to excess light or moisture.

Drugs should not be transferred from one container to another, and containers must be clearly labelled.

> *An individual patient's response to any drug may be at variance with intended/expected effects*

The physical state of the patient such as the age, weight or metabolic rate may affect the response to any drug.

Any history of allergy or sensitivity, should be reported prior to administration of the initial dose of a drug.

The presence of side effects or toxic effects should be reported prior to the administration of any further doses of any prescribed drug.

The effect of one drug may differ in the presence of another drug or substance.

Pharmacists, drug manufacturers or poisons centres, should be contacted as necessary.

Effectiveness of all drugs should be evaluated in order that changes in prescription may be made.

> *Drug therapy may form part of long-term or life-long treatment*

An objective of nursing is to help each patient, where appropriate, to manage and administer his own drugs.

Each patient has his own needs for explanation and support with respect to his drug regime.

The patient and his relatives must be given enough information to understand the drug regime and why the drug is being taken.

The patient and his relatives must be allowed to gain confidence in administering the drugs independently.

The patient undergoing long-term drug therapy may need to carry pertinent information with him at all times.

Regular monitoring of drug therapy may be required.

> *An element of error is a possibility in all human activity.*
> *Elimination of errors is dependent upon the*
> *nurse's constant vigilance and attention to detail*

Experience has shown that it is all too easy for a moments inattention, a momentary distraction, tiredness or pressure of work, to cause a wrong drug or an incorrect amount to be given to a patient.

If an error is made, it should be reported immediately and help sought from nursing and medical colleagues to safeguard the patient.

Further reading

Bickerton J., Sampson A.C.M. & Boylan A. (1979) *Nursing: Theory and Practice,* pp 152–154. McGraw-Hill (UK) Ltd, London. (Helping patients avoid injection hazards.)

Oxfordshire Health Authority (1985) *Drugs Code of Practice for Nurses.* (All nurses, nursing students, medical and pharmaceutical staff are given a copy of this code.)

Drug Administration—a nursing responsibility (1980), pp 1–10. Royal College of Nursing, London.

Pain Control

Pain is a total experience with physical, mental, and emotional components.

Pain is unique to the individual—a subjective experience. Pain cannot be seen, is difficult to describe or recall precisely and is problematic in evaluation. Pain, therefore, must be what the individual says it is, occurs when and where he says it occurs, and hurts as much as he describes.

> *Pain is a physiological mechanism, often protective,*
> *since it signals damage to body tissues*

The pain threshold is the first point at which pain is felt by an individual.

Pain has a definite pattern related to time, intensity, duration and type.

Acute pain is short term, and has a forseeable end despite its possible severity. Pain prompts the individual to seek a cause and immediate relief.

Chronic pain is prolonged, altering the quality of the person's life, physically, and emotionally. It reminds the individual constantly of his health status, and may lead to introspection and social isolation.

Pain theories include:

- Specificity theory—certain sense organs are specially adapted to detect and transmit the presence of painful stimuli.
- Pattern theory—the pattern of nerve impulses and summation of input from a particular body area triggers cerebral interpretation of pain stimuli.
- Gate-control theory—the dorsal horn of the spinal cord acts as a gate mechanism, allowing increase or decrease in the flow of pain impulses.
- Descending impulses from the brain may trigger release of endorphins, opiate-like substances, in afferent nerves thus inhibiting pain sensation transmission.

Damaged tissues for example sunburnt skin, are more sensitive to painful stimuli.

The area of the body surrounding damaged tissue is often more sensitive to pain than normal tissue.

Severe pain in one area of the body may detract from perception of more moderate pain sensation in other areas. For example a headache may be superceded by the pain from a scalded hand.

Physical manifestations of pain include:

- pallor, low blood pressure, tachycardia, muscle guarding
- restlessness, altered consciousness and collapse may occur as pain intensity increases.

> *Pain perception and expression may be influenced by psychological and emotional factors*

Anticipation of pain produces anxiety.

Anxiety and fear intensify pain sensation. However if pain is totally unanticipated it can appear more intense.

Tiredness, depression and isolation tend to increase sensitivity to painful stimuli.

Emotional states such as extreme excitement, euphoria, or profound shock may decrease pain perception.

Meaningful pain may be more easily tolerated. For example in childbirth, war wounds or perhaps if pain is seen as punishment for past misdeeds it may appear less severe.

Involvement in activities which are intrinsically interesting and motivating may diminish pain perception.

> **Pain perception and expression may be influenced by
> cultural and environmental factors**

Age may affect pain expression. For example, whilst a child may openly express pain, the adult may have learned to modify or limit expression.

Expression of pain is partly determined by early experience and cultural expectations. However the same individual may respond variously under differing circumstances.

Life circumstances may affect pain perception and tolerance. For example, living conditions, the amount of environmental 'noise' or the presence of anxiety-provoking factors such as financial difficulties.

The attitudes of others may affect pain expression.

> **Assessment must include the patient's subjective impressions
> of his pain as well as objective observations**

NB *The pattern of pain is not necessarily related to the disease process.*

The nurse must be aware of her own bias and values about pain.

The quality, location, intensity, time and duration of pain are important for diagnosis and treatment. Factors which precipitate or alleviate the pain should be noted.

Pain may be manifest non-verbally in facial expression, posture, skin colour and mood state.

Assessment tools include pain scales, body outline charts, and questionnaires. These provide a written record and facilitate continuity of care.

> *Interventions to ease pain must include*
> *psychological and physical elements*

Nursing intervention includes:

Reasonable, clear explanations, which may limit anxiety.

Establishing rapport, remaining calm, listening without judging.

Comfort measures such as cool, crease-free linen or limiting environmental noise.

Ensuring that physiological needs are met and problems such as nausea or constipation are prevented.

Changing the position of the patient to relieve sensitive areas.

Physical support for painful areas, such as a bandage to support a limb, a hand to hold a wound.

The application of local warmth, such as a kaolin poultice or heat pad.

The application of ice packs, or cold compresses to hot, inflamed areas.

Facilitating diversional therapies such as reading, listening to the radio, and involving the occupational therapist where appropriate.

Ensuring adequate rest, relaxation and sleep.

Regular evaluation of the effectiveness of prescribed analgesia, observation for side effects, and communication of findings.

NB *A patient who demands analgesia is unlikely to be addicted. It may be that he cannot rely on you to respond to his needs and keep him pain free. In anticipation of returning pain he demands analgesia.*

The nurse must be open to the inclusion of alternative therapies to reduce suffering, such as:

- progressive relaxation exercises,
- massage,
- meditation or hypnotherapy,
- acupuncture.

Medical interventions include:

- prescription of primary and/or secondary analgesics,
- transcutaneous nerve stimulation therapy,
- surgical intervention with severence of nerves to affected areas,
- the use of anaesthetic agents, such as epidural or local injections.

Further reading

Anon. (1980) Pain relief—the nurse's role. *Nursing Times* **76**(24): 1052–1054.

Bond M.R. (1979) *Pain: its Nature, Analysis and Treatment*. Churchill Livingstone, Edinburgh.

Condon P. (1985) Pain control therapeutics. *Professional Nurse*, October 1985.

McCaffey M. (1983) *Nursing the Patient in Pain*. Harper and Rowe, London.

Twycross R.G. Principles and practice of pain relief in terminal cancer. Sir Michael Sobell House, Churchill Hospital, Oxford.

Stress

Stress is experienced when physical, mental, or emotional stimuli, as perceived by the individual, cannot be easily tolerated.

Personal characteristics and emotions determine how each individual interprets physical, mental and emotional stressors. Past experience, the physical state at the time, the number of stressors, and the resource systems possessed by the individual, influence how he will cope. Individuals must develop coping mechanisms to deal with stress. Coping is defined as dealing successfully with an event and gaining control over it.

> *A variety of factors are likely to*
> *produce stress in patients*

Examples include:
- a strange environment, unfamiliar surroundings, or disorientation.
- the loss of personal identity produced when clothing is removed, time schedules are imposed by others or control of one's own environment is affected.
- the use of medical terminology which may be unfamiliar to the patient.
- the need to be dependent upon others for physiological needs, such as food, toilet facilities, or even oxygen.
- isolation from others necessitated by such things as barrier nursing and during X-ray procedures.
- separation from loved ones.
- excessive interpersonal contact. For example exposure, in a short time span, to various members of the multidisciplinary team can be very demanding.
- excessive or unfamiliar noise levels, or the strange smells which may be encountered in the clinical environment.

> *Nurses, like any other people may*
> *be subject to excess stress*

Examples include:
- factors inherent in any occupation, such as organizational change, long working hours, too little or too much work or too little time to complete workload.
- emotional involvement with patients, especially the dying, or those with distressing symptoms or diseases.
- interpersonal or communication difficulties within the multi-disciplinary team.
- the conflict between idealism and reality.

> *Stress produces physical manifestations*

The heart rate and blood pressure rise.

Muscle tone increases.

Pupillary dilation heightens visual acuity, however the perceptual field is decreased, since attention is focused on the stressful stimulus. For example, the slightest noise will startle a stressed person.

Tension headaches, sleeplessness or restlessness may occur.

Disease processes, such as hypertension or peptic ulcer may be precipitated.

> **Stress induces psychological defence mechanisms**
> **which may help the person to cope,**
> **these were described by Freud as follows**

Rationalization — finding an acceptable reason for feeling stressed, such as pressure of work.

Denial/disbelief — on hearing a diagnosis, for example, the patient may suggest that he is being confused with someone else.

Displacement — directing hostile feelings about the stressor at someone or something else. For example, a patient in pain may shout at the nurse.

Repression — faced with chronic illness the patient may not perceive a need to change his lifestyle.

> **Understanding the stress response**
> **may assist in managing stress**

The individual needs to identify what activates the stress response.

Determining when stress occurs may be important in its management.

Physical responses should be noted. For example:
- are the muscles tensed?
- is concentration or memory impaired?
- is the heart rate raised?

Subjective feelings should be examined.

Behavioural changes should be noted.

> *Avoidance or reduction strategies may be utilized*
> *to offset the effects of stress*

Individual strengths and talents should be identified and cultivated.

Making time for recreation, or physical activities, may reduce the perception of stressful stimuli.

Improving self-perception abilities by drawing on the skills of a counsellor or psychotherapist where necessary, may assist.

Interventions such as assertiveness training, or bio-feedback techniques should be considered.

Spiritual support may bring benefits for some individuals.

Techniques such as meditation or progressive relaxation may be utilized.

> *Patient stress may be reduced*
> *by effective nursing interventions*

Existing coping strategies should be supported.

Accurate information and adequate explanations should be given.

The patient should be involved in decision-making, choice and control in aspects of care being facilitated.

'Meaningful others' should be involved in the patient's care if this reduces stress.

Expression of feelings should be allowed, for example, crying may relieve the tension of stress.

Adequate rest and sleep should be facilitated.

Prescribed therapies, such as the use of night sedation or anxiolytic drugs, should be regularly evaluated.

Diversional activities, and complementary therapies such as massage or aromatherapy, may prove beneficial in reducing the stress response.

Further reading

Davitz L.J. & Davitz R.J. (1975) How do nurses feel when patients suffer? *American Journal of Nursing* **75:** 1505–1510.

Freud A. (1966) *The Ego and Mechanisms of Defence.* Hogarth Press, London.

Parker K.R. (1980) Occupational stress among student nurses. *Nursing Times* **76:** 113–119.

Selye H. (1956/1976) *The Stress of Life.* McGraw-Hill, Maidenhead.

Spielberger C. (1979) *Understanding Stress and Anxiety.* Harper and Rowe, London.

Control of Infection

The fundamental aim of infection control is to avoid the transfer of potential pathogenic micro-organisms from one person, or site, to another.

Micro-organisms are everywhere in the environment, the majority are harmless to humans, whilst some are beneficial. All need an environment in which they can grow and multiply.

Micro-organisms include bacteria, viruses, fungi, protozoa and helminths. Harmful micro-organisms are called pathogens.

Pathogenic organisms produce infection if the right environment is provided.

Normal body structure and activities provide the individual with considerable protection against infection

---

The body possesses, in health, its own microbial flora—these are helpful organisms which assist the body with normal functioning.

The intact skin is an effective barrier against the entry of micro-organisms.

By their action, the mucous membranes and cilia of the respiratory tract, assist in the removal of inhaled micro-organisms.

Body fluids may contain antibacterial substances such as lysozyme in tears.

Gastro-intestinal tract secretions such as hydrochloric acid, and digestive enzymes, afford protection through a bactericidal action.

Normal flora of the vagina produce acid secretions which deter infective organisms.

The process of inflammation is designed to localize invading micro-organisms and augment the phagocytic/destructive action of polymorphonuclear leucocytes and macrophages.

The reticulo-endothelial immune system offers further protection against certain micro-organisms.

> *Infection implies that micro-organisms have overcome normal body defenses and have entered the body, grown and multiplied*

The number and virulence of the organisms may determine the degree of infection. Virulence relates to the ability of the organism to survive, multiply and damage the person's tissues.

The degree of infection also depends upon the resistance of the person. This is determined by factors such as age, nutrition, hygiene status, occupation, the presence of concomitant disease processes, and the state of the reticulo-endothelial immune system.

The chain of infection

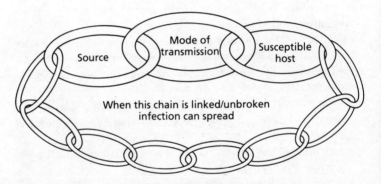

The source can be animate or inanimate.

The mode of transmission may include:

- person to person.
- contact between a person and a contaminated surface or object.
- airborne infection including organisms exhaled in droplets from the respiratory tract.
- insect or animal vectors.

A susceptible host is one in whom resistance to infection is lowered.

> *Infection is controlled by breaking any of the links in the chain*

The Source—is the reservoir of infection.

Identification and destruction of the causative organism is the first step toward control.

Methods used to destroy micro-organisms include sterilization and gamma irradiation.

Staff with infection should take precautionary measures.

Statutory provisions exist for the control of pests, provision of clean food and water, and air, and the notification of certain diseases.

Susceptible host

Attention to personal hygiene, diet, exercise, sleep and rest may improve individual resistance to infection.

Vaccination and immunization will increase resistance to specific organisms.

Certain patients do not have an infective disease but are extremely susceptible to infection. For example, the immunosuppressed patient may need to have physical barriers established to protect them from extrinsic commensals and pathogens.

Transmission

Barriers between micro-organisms and the potential host will interrupt or break the chain at this point and therefore prevent the spread of infection.

Handwashing and careful drying is a most important activity in preventing the transmission of infection.

A high standard of environmental cleanliness deters spread of infection which requires the co-ordination of many services.

Cleaning and disinfecting of the physical surroundings, including equipment used for patients must be carried out regularly.

Clean equipment and services should be available to each individual patient.

Clean and dirty supplies should be clearly separated.

Clean and dirty techniques should be performed separately.

Correct disposal of waste is essential.

Many micro-organisms are carried in air, therefore:
- good ventilation of patient areas is essential.
- patients should have sufficient personal space.
- 'through traffic' in critical areas should be limited.
- inappropriate activity and movement of equipment such as curtains or bedlinen should be avoided.

Segregation of an infected patient may be necessay to protect other people from the micro-organisms causing the disease, this may be in a restricted area where physical barriers such as doors, face masks, gowns or gloves are used.

Notice of isolation should be clearly visible and *all* staff informed.

Colour coded cards are used in many hospitals to denote those patients requiring isolation nursing. These guide the nurse in the specific actions she takes for individual patients. Facsimiles are reproduced here.

PATIENT IN ISOLATION

ALL VISITORS must report to the nurses' station before entering this room.

BLOOD AND BODY FLUIDS PRECAUTIONS

1 HANDS. All staff and visitors must wash hands before and after attending the patient. An alcoholic hand disinfectant is acceptable for socially clean hands.

2 MASKS not indicated.

3 GOWNS OR PLASTIC APRONS to be worn if handling infected material.

4 GLOVES to be worn when handling infected material.

5 BLOOD AND BODY FLUID SPILLS must be promptly cleaned up with a solution of sodium hypochlorite diluted 1:10 with water.

6 ALL NEEDLE STICK INJURIES should be reported immediately.

PATIENTS REQUIRING
BLOOD AND BODY FLUIDS ISOLATION

All patients with drainage of infected fluid from the chest and abdomen, where the infecting organism is potentially hazardous to other patients.

HEPATITIS B AND ACQUIRED
IMMUNE DEFICIENCY SYNDROME (AIDS)

Risks can only be defined by laboratory investigation. Isolation may not always be necessary. Seek further advice from the virology laboratory.

It may be necessary to take frequent specimens to establish presence of infective organisms.

Isolation may be discontinued on laboratory clearance. If in doubt seek medical advice.

SPECIAL PRECAUTIONS

1 BLOOD AND BODY FLUID SPILLAGES must be properly cleaned up with a solution of sodium hypochlorite diluted 1:10 in water, obtainable from pharmacy.

2 ALL NEEDLE STICK INJURIES should be reported immediately.

3 INFECTED MATERIAL must be double bagged in yellow plastic bags for incineration. Material from highly infectious patients will require rapid disposal.

4 TERMINAL DISINFECTION OF ROOM after discharge of infected patients is necessary. Follow current procedure.

PATIENT IN ISOLATION

VISITING RESTRICTED TO ESSENTIAL PERSONNEL otherwise at the discretion of the nurse in charge.
ALL VISITORS must report to the nurses' station before entering this room.

PRECAUTIONS FOR PROTECTIVE ISOLATION

1 HANDS. All staff and visitors must wash hands before and
after attending the patient. An alcoholic hand disinfectant is
acceptable for socially clean hands.
2 MASKS to be worn only if specified.
3 GLOVES not indicated.
4 GOWNS OR PLASTIC APRONS to be worn.

PATIENTS REQUIRING PROTECTIVE ISOLATION

1 NEUTROPAENIC
2 IMMUNOSUPPRESSED
3 EXTENSIVE BURNS
4 NEONATES REQUIRING SPECIAL VENTILATION
NB PROCEDURE FOR TERMINAL DISINFECTION OF
   ROOM TO BE FOLLOWED PRIOR TO PATIENT'S
   ADMISSION.

SPECIAL PRECAUTIONS

1 INDIVIDUALIZED NURSING CARE
2 MEDICAL STAFF RESTRICTED TO ESSENTIAL
   PERSONNEL ONLY
3 OTHER VISITORS TO BE KEPT TO A MINIMUM

PATIENT IN ISOLATION

ALL VISITORS must report to the nurses' station before entering this room.

RESPIRATORY PRECAUTIONS

1 HANDS. All staff and visitors must wash their hands before and after attending the patient. An alcoholic hand disinfectant is acceptable for socially clean hands.

2 MASKS only to be worn by staff in close contact with patient.

3 GOWNS OR PLASTIC APRONS to be worn when handling infected material.

4 GLOVES to be worn when handling infected material.

PATIENTS REQUIRING ISOLATION FOR RESPIRATORY INFECTIONS

1 Severe lung infections
2 Some viral pneumonias
3 Staphylococcal pneumonia
4 Some viral diseases common to children:
Measles, Chicken Pox,
Herpes, Mumps,
Respiratory syncytial virus
5 Mycoplasma infections
6 Whooping cough

7 Productive cough. This may include tuberculosis but patients should be transferred to care of the chest unit at the Churchill Hopital as soon as possible
8 Meningococcal meningitis until initial treatment is effective

Not all patients with pneumonia require isolation. If in doubt seek medical advice. Isolation may be discontinued on bacteriological clearance.

NB It is important to obtain 3 sputum specimens as soon as possible after admission or onset of respiratory infection.

SPECIAL PRECAUTIONS

1 Infected material to be double bagged using yellow plastic sacks for disposal by incineration.
Material from highly infected patients will require rapid disposal. See clinical waste disposal procedure.

2 Terminal disinfection of room is necessary. See current procedure.

PATIENT IN ISOLATION

ALL VISITORS must report to the nurses' station before entering this room.

ENTERIC PRECAUTIONS

1 HANDS. All staff and visitors must wash hands before and after attending the patient. An alcoholic hand disinfectant is acceptable for socially clean hands.

2 MASKS not indicated.

3 GOWNS OR PLASTIC APRONS to be worn if soiling is likely.

4 GLOVES to be worn when handling infected material.

SEE PROCEDURE FOR DISPOSAL OF ARTICLES CONTAMINATED WITH INFECTED MATERIAL.

PATIENTS REQUIRING ISOLATION FOR ENTERIC INFECTIONS

1 SALMONELLA   **3** ACUTE GASTRO-ENTERITIS

2 DYSENTRY   **4** INFECTIOUS HEPATITIS

All patients admitted with diarrhoea of unknown origin must be isolated.

Isolation is not always necessary when a patient is producing a formed stool.

Isolation may be discontinued on bacteriological clearance.

NB It is important to send a specimen of faeces for bacteriological investigation as soon as possible after onset of diarrhoea.

SPECIAL PRECAUTIONS

1 Wherever possible, A SINGLE ROOM with a separate facility for disposal of excreta i.e. own toilet or commode.

2 THE BEDPAN MACERATOR OR WASHER/DISINFECTOR must be carefully disinfected (inner and outer surfaces) after disposal of infected excreta.

3 INFECTED MATERIAL must be double bagged in yellow plastic bags for disposal by incineration. Material from highly infectious patients will require rapid disposal by incineration.

3 CROCKERY AND CUTLERY should follow normal washing up procedure for non-infected patients.

5 TERMINAL DISINFECTION of room after discharge of infected patients is necessary, following current procedure.

Further reading

Gibson J.M. (1979) *Modern Microbiology and Pathology for Nurses.* Blackwell Scientific Publications, Oxford.

Maurer I.M. (1979) *Hospital Hygiene.* Edward Arnold, London.

Meers P.D. & Stronge J.L. (1978) Hospitals should do the sick no harm. Parts 1–6. *Nursing Times Supplement.*

Taylor L.J. An evaluation of handwashing techniques. *Nursing Times Supplement* **74**(2) January 12: 54–55 and (3) January 19: 108–110.

The Principles of Asepsis

Asepsis is the state of being completely free from all living pathogenic organisms.

Asepsis is essential:

- when there is injury undermining the integrity of the skin;
- when the skin is to be incised or penetrated during surgical operations, or procedures such as bone marrow biopsy, or injections;
- when a sterile body cavity will be entered or penetrated during a procedure, such as abdominal paracentesis, chest aspiration, lumbar puncture;
- when body defences are undermined by illness, increasing the risk of concomitant infections.

It is neither possible, nor desirable, for a nurse to memorize a set of rules for each and every situation which might be encountered. The objective of aseptic practice is to avoid adding micro-organisms to any site where they may cause damage, and to maintain aseptic sites such that the environment is rendered unfavourable to micro-organisms.

Any nurses with a known or suspected infection should not carry out care requiring aseptic practice.

Skin is unsterile and carries micro-organisms. The nurse's hands *must* therefore be thoroughly washed and dried prior to any treatment requiring aseptic practice.

- This renders the hands socially clean *but not aseptic*.
- Sterile forceps can now be used to manipulate other sterile equipment.
- Subsequent hand contact with an area or object which is not sterile, contaminates the hands and may necessitate repeat handwashing.
- To obviate the need for frequent handwashing during any treatment, all necessary equipment should be available and conveniently situated at the outset, and the patient adequately prepared. This includes explanation to gain co-operation, administration of prescribed analgesia if necessary and careful positioning for optimal patient comfort.

121

> *A sterile object or area becomes contaminated when contact*
> *occurs with a wet surface, or liquid from a wet surface*

When washing the hands prior to, and during any treatment, wet hands should be held above elbow level to prevent water from the arms running back over socially clean hands.

The hands must be thoroughly dried after washing to reduce the possibility of contact of sterile objects with moisture.

A sterile, porous material will serve as a barrier between an unsterile surface and a sterile object such as a trolley top, or surface *only* if the material is dry.

Wrappers of packs from manufacturers or sterile supplies departments should be checked. If wet, the contents must not be used.

If lotions are to be used as part of treatment they must be sterile and bactericidal.

Clean, dry wounds should never be made moist by the use of cleansing lotion.

> *If a sterile object touches an unsterile object or area*
> *contamination occurs*

No sterile material should be touched directly by hand—forceps or surgical gloves must be used.

Packs from manufacturers or sterile supplies departments should be checked for damage which would allow the contents to be contaminated from the exterior. Damaged packs must be discarded.

Wherever possible sterile objects should be kept above waist level to increase visibility and lessen the risk of accidental contact with unsterile objects.

The sterile area should be continually in view in order to lessen the possibility of unintentional contamination.

> *A sterile object or area becomes contaminated*
> *when micro-organisms are transported to it*
> *by air currents or gravity*

Air currents must be kept to a minimum by avoiding unnecessary movement of equipment and people, ensuring that bedmaking, ward cleaning and closure of bed curtains is completed prior to commencing the treatment reduces the risk.

Aseptic sites should be exposed for as short a time as possible. Correct preparation of the patient and equipment should facilitate this.

'Clean' wounds or treatment should receive attention before 'dirty' (infected) wounds, or treatments.

To avoid adding micro-organisms when treating a break in the continuity of the skin, cleaning should be from the least contaminated area to the most contaminated.

Excessive talking is discouraged. Droplets of moisture, saliva or sputum may contaminate the area.

Similarly, laughing, coughing and sneezing will introduce micro-organisms into the environment.

The nurse should not reach across the sterile area. Micro-organisms from her body or clothing may fall onto the area.

Because there is always a chance that micro-organisms carried by air currents may have contaminated sterile equipment, once opened, the contents of a sterile pack should not be used for any other aseptic technique.

> *An object or area is either* **sterile** *or it is* **contaminated**.
> *It cannot be almost sterile.*
> *If there is any doubt consider the object contaminated.*
> *The provision of a safe environment is paramount.*
> *This means patient safety*

Requirements for basic aseptic techniques

Dressing pack	Adhesive tape
Ancillary packs as required	Scissors
Skin cleansing lotions	Disposable bag for used dressings
Dressing solutions as required	CSSD disposable bag.

Guidelines for specific practices requiring an aseptic technique

Abdominal paracentesis—care of the patient

Abdominal paracentesis is the insertion of a cannula into the peritoneal space:

- to facilitate the withdrawal of fluid from the abdominal cavity to relieve pressure,
- for diagnostic purposes,
- to provide a route for the administration of drugs such as cytotoxic agents.

The principles of asepsis and control of infection apply.

The patient is placed in the most comfortable position which will also achieve optimum drainage (generally sitting up well supported with pillows).

If fluid is being withdrawn the amount to drain must be ascertained from the doctor, and the rate of flow regulated accordingly—a corset may need to be applied to the abdomen and tightened from time to time to assist compression and thus drainage.

Observation should include pulse rate, peripheral circulation status, colour and skin condition because of the possibility of shock occurring when fluid is withdrawn.

Whilst the cannula remains in position and draining, the entry site is observed for signs of infection.

On removal of the cannula a sterile occlusive dressing is applied.

NB *The bladder should be emptied prior to insertion of the cannula.*

Requirements

The appropriate CSSD pack
Local anaesthetic, syringes, needles
Skin cleansing lotions including povidone iodine
Sterile specimen bottles
Adhesive tape
Drainage bag
Regulator clip
Abdominal corset
Receptacle for used materials.

Guidelines for care of the patient having a lumbar puncture

This is the simplest method of obtaining access to the sub-arachnoid space and, may be performed:

- to obtain cerebro-spinal fluid for examination, and to estimate its pressure,
- for the relief of intracranial pressure and the removal of toxic inflammatory or other irritative substances in the cerebro-spinal fluid,
- to introduce therapeutic substances or local anaesthetic into the subarachnoid space or dyes for radiographic purposes.

The procedure is carried out by a doctor with a nurse assisting.

The principles of asepsis and control of infection apply.

Sedation may be given before the procedure if necessary.

The patient assumes the lateral position—the greatest possible degree of flexion of the lumbar spine is required to facilitate insertion of the spinal needle. This is achieved by the patient drawing the knees to the chin, the nurse assisting the patient to maintain this position.

If specimens of cerebro-spinal fluid are withdrawn they are collected in sterile containers and labelled in the order in which they were obtained, prior to being sent to the laboratory.

After the procedure, when the needle is withdrawn a sterile occlusive dressing is applied.

The patient is advised to lie flat for between 6 and 24 hours, in order to prevent development of a headache.

NB *Observation for changes in the level of consciousness should be made during, and following this procedure.*

Requirements

A basic wound dressing pack
Spinal needles and Greenfield manometer
Skin cleansing lotions including povidone iodine
Local anaesthetic, syringes, needles
Sterile specimen containers
Adhesive tape for occlusive dressing.

Guidelines for chest aspiration

NB *The co-operation of the patient is essential in this procedure. To prevent the aspirating needle puncturing the visceral pleura the patient is asked to remain quite still during the procedure and not to cough without warning, preferably not to cough at all. Analgesia and cough linctus may therefore need to be given prior to the procedure.*

The principles of asepsis and control of infection apply.

The patient sits upright and leans forward since the doctor requires easy access to the posterior chest wall.

The most recent chest X-ray should be available to aid the doctor in selection of an appropriate site for insertion of the aspiration needle.

The main role of the nurse is to support the patient physically and psychologically, and to observe the pulse rate, respiration, colour of the skin and mucous membranes in order to detect respiratory or cardiovascular problems. The presence of chest pain must also be noted and reported to the doctor.

Resuscitation equipment should be available throughout the procedure.

On removal of the aspiration needle a sterile occlusive dressing is applied.

Observation of pulse rate, respiration and colour should continue until stability of the patient's condition is assured.

Any aspirate specimens should be clearly labelled and sent to the laboratory.

Requirements

Patient's X-rays
The appropriate CSSD pack
Skin cleansing lotions plus povidone iodine
Local anaesthetic, syringes, needles
Sterile specimen bottles
Measuring jug (sterile)
Adhesive tape
Receptacle for used materials
Resuscitation equipment.

Further reading

Du Gas B.W. (1977) *Introduction to patient care*, 3rd edition, Ch. 22, pp 415–432. W.B. Saunders & Company, Philadelphia.

Hall S.E. (1978) Caring for wounds. *Nursing Mirror Supplement* **146**(10) March 9 ix, xi, xiii.

Record Keeping

Recording is the communication in writing of essential facts in order to maintain a continuous history of events over a period of time.
Reporting is the communication of information to another individual or group and may be written or oral.

> *The main purpose of patient records is to provide a written account of the data that have been gathered about the patient; and about the management of the patient*

All information gathered for record purposes should be regarded as confidential between the patient and the professionals caring for him.

Although the record is the property of the hospital or health authority it is increasingly felt nowadays that the patient has a right of access to the information contained therein.

The data serve as a means of communication among those whose talents are directed towards the patient's care.

The data serve as a basis on which the care team plans the diagnostic and therapeutic regime.

Patient records provide a permanent account for future reference, as well as for teaching and research purposes.

The records are admissable as evidence in a court of law.

Patient records may be required for use in the collection of statistics.

Components of patient's records

Different records and report forms are kept by the various health units. However, although the number and design may vary there are certain commonalities among most records kept in this country.

Nursing notes

A patient assessment is made based on an agreed model of nursing.

Patient problems are determined from data gathered during patient assessment.

A plan of care is devised which includes diagnostic, therapeutic and educational aspects of care related to each problem.

Care is evaluated against the previously determined patient outcome for each problem.

The nursing record demonstrates that care is systematically planned and is not a haphazard series of events.

Nursing records help to maintain continuity of care and provide a means of communication between nurses and others.

Medical records

Most health care units have an admission sheet on which are recorded basic biographical and some social data about the patient. The data are usually accurate and can be transcribed to other records when necessary.

The history sheet is generally completed by the doctor when the patient is admitted to the unit. This is a record of the personal and medical history of the patient.

Information from other sources regarding the condition of the patient is included in the medical record.

Included in the medical records are sheets used to store investigation and pathological reports.

Consent forms for medical interventions will be kept with these records.

The medical notes provide a valuable source of information for the nurse in the development of her plan of care.

Patient charts

Most health care units will have recognized printed charts for record purposes, these may include:
- medicine sheet, used by doctors to prescribe therapeutic regimes.
- observation charts, used by nurses to record measurable information about the patient.
- charts used to record details of surgical intervention and anaesthestic administration.

Guidelines for record keeping

All recordings should be accurate and truthful.

Omission of a recording is as inaccurate as an incorrect recording.

Narrative recordings should be concise and specific.

All recordings should be complete and legible.

Erasures are not allowed—errors should be crossed through with a single line and the correct information inserted.

Ink must be used, and all entries dated and signed.

Different coloured inks may be used in nursing records to denote different time periods, for example black ink may be used by day staff for writing reports, red ink for the night staff report.

Correct spelling is essential to avoid errors of interpretation.

The frequency with which recordings are made should be decided by the individual unit, and will vary according to the rate of change in the patient's condition.

The minimum of abbreviations should be used.

(We recognize that abbreviations have a place in record keeping, but there are inherent dangers in their use.)

It is the professional's responsibility in any clinical area to decide the acceptable abbreviations, but these must be communicated to all others in the area.

If you use an abbreviation are you sure it is unambiguous? Can your communication be understood by the next person to read it?

Further reading

Du Gas B.W. (1983) *Introduction to Patient Care*, 4th edition, Ch. 12, pp 217–228. Saunders International, Philadelphia.

Kings Fund (1979) *A Handbook for Nurse to Nurse Reporting*. Kings Fund Centre.

Open University (1984) *A Systematic Approach to Patient Care*. Open University Press, Milton Keynes.

Part III
Professional and Organizational Aspects of Care

Professional and Ethical Issues

Every profession is based on a code of ethics which places positive values on the purposes and activities of the members of that profession. This code commits the professional to certain values of service to others above those of income, power and prestige.

Professional issues

> *The nurse is morally and legally accountable
> to the patient/client for her professional practice*

The nurse is responsible both for the physical care she gives, and the
advice she offers in the course of her duties.

The nurse has a duty of care towards the patient/client so that
unreasonable risks are not taken and the forseeable consequences
are weighed.

The law requires that the nurse takes every reasonable opportunity to
maintain and improve professional knowledge and competence
commensurate with qualifications, position and experience.

The nurse respects and holds in confidence all personal information
obtained in the course of practice, unless consent for disclosure is
obtained from the patient/client, or the law so requires.

> *Health authorities have a responsibility
> toward the staff in their employ*

The health authority should ensure that staff are properly qualified,
and adequately instructed, in order to care for those in their
charge.

The nurse should have a contract of service clearly identifying line
accountability within the organization.

The health authority has vicarious responsibility on the part of its
staff, and is liable for damages awarded against them.

In cases of litigation against staff, the health authority is expected to
undertake defence of nursing staff.

However, the authority has the right, in common law, to claim
indemnity against an individual proven negligent, and it is likely
that disciplinary action will be taken.

Guidelines for maintaining safe practice

The nurse must maintain individual competence by observation, investigation, and continued study.

The nurse uses individual competence as a criterion for accepting delegated responsibilities.

If new work is accepted, the nurse must agree that it is a reasonable commitment, and that proper safeguards are taken.

If the nurse delegates work she must ensure that staff are not asked to perform tasks for which they are not fitted, or from which they are prohibited by legal enactment.

The nurse should acknowledge any limitations of her competence, and should not accept responsibility for work she does not feel prepared to undertake.

Student nurses bear a measure of responsibility, and will be judged according to their stage in training.

Good communication skills and accurate record keeping are an important adjunct to safe practice.

The nurse should be aware of what constitutes a safe environment for the patient/client, and for other members of the caring team, and make known any circumstances which could mitigate against safe standards.

Ethical issues

The nurse will face many, and complex, ethical dilemmas in the course of her work. A dilemma has been defined as a situation requiring a choice between what seem to be two equally desirable or undesirable alternatives.

In making ethical decisions:
- Each individual must think through the dilemma for themselves, but, it may help in reaching a decision, to think *about* others, and *with* others.
- All relevant considerations must be identified, and critically examined.
- Asking the right questions may enable the right decision to be made for that individual.
- A person's religious, cultural, and philosophical beliefs may influence decision making.
- In an ethical situation there is not likely to be an absolute answer.
- Decisions should be based on what is right for the individual patient/client, and/or his family.

Ethical considerations can be discussed under a variety of headings, and we have offered just a few examples of the sorts of dilemmas occurring almost daily in nursing which may provide topics for thought or discussion.

> *There are some situations where the nurse may have to decide whether she should risk losing a patient's trust by disclosing information she has been offered in confidence*

Examples include:
- The breaking of confidence, where the nurse considers that disclosure would be beneficial to the welfare of the patient.
- The breaking of confidence in giving information to legal agencies, for example when there is a threat to life.
- Betrayal of the confidence of a colleague where the nurse believes that professional practice may be jeopardized.

The rights, well-being and safety of the individual may be determining factors in arriving at a decision.

> *Where two or more professionals are*
> *involved in the care of one patient*
> *differences of opinion may arise*

Examples include:
- The continuation or withdrawal of particular treatments.
- Truthfulness in the giving or witholding of information from the patient or his family, or such things as the giving of placebos instead of actual medication.
- The expansion of nursing knowledge, and the wish for autonomy, which may produce tensions between nurse and doctor if lines of communication are not clear.

It should always be borne in mind that sound decisions cannot be made without the knowledge and experience of all the care team. However, the nurse should remember that the patient is her primary focus of care.

> *Philosophical beliefs may involve the*
> *nurse in conscientious refusal of care*

Examples include:
- Involvement in medical research—the search for knowledge with no clearly identified beneficial patient outcome, may appear unjustified. However, the need to expand knowledge to improve care should always be considered.
- In a patient suffering from a terminal illness, the nurse may feel it detrimental to the patient or his family to implement resuscitative measures.
- Personal beliefs may leave the nurse feeling that she cannot assist with the act of abortion, or the giving of contraceptive advice.

The extent to which involvement in care would jeopardize personal integrity must be weighed against the emotions or sanctions which might follow refusal.

> *The need for health care requires that certain services are provided, resource allocation may therefore raise ethical questions*

Examples include:

- The inequality in health service provision which results in differing mortality and morbidity rates in separate geographical areas, and between social classes.
- The funding of particular medical specialities, which may appear to be at the expense of others.
- Individual care areas such as the community, a hospital, or a specific patient care unit, having to compete actively for scant resources.

Nurses have social as well as individual obligations.

The code of the International Council of Nurses states, 'The nurse shares with other citizens the responsibility for initiating and supporting action to meet the health and social needs of the public'.

Further reading

Baly M.E. (1984) *Professional Responsibility*, 2nd edition. John Wiley & Son, Chichester.

Benjamin M. & Curtis J. (1981) *Ethics in Nursing*. Oxford University Press, Oxford.

DHSS (1977) *The Extending Role of the Clinical Nurse*. DHSS Publication.

Du Gas B.W. (1983) *Introduction to Patient Care*, 4th edition. Saunders International, Philadelphia.

Royal College of Nursing (1978) *The Duties and Position of the Nurse*. Royal College of Nursing Publication.

Young A.P. (1981) *Legal Problems in Nursing Practice*. Harper & Row, London.

Decision Making

Problem solving is the crux of professional practice, and decision making the hallmark of a profession.

In nursing, problem solving and decision making are the central core of planned patient care.

The nurse as a decision maker

The introduction of new ways of organizing and delivering nursing, so that the total care of an individual patient is the responsibility of one nurse, pre-supposes that the nurse will make intelligent, independent decisions, about complex patient care problems, relating to the delivery of health services.

It has been said that the ability to reason systematically is a basic necessity for any manager who hopes to manage well. All nurses are managers, and intrinsic in that role are complex problem-solving situations. The multiple needs of patients, the demands of the health care system for continued nursing services, and the many emergencies that confront nurses, require them to act decisively. Unless a systematic, reasoned approach is employed, time and energy may be wasted in making decisions which may prove ineffective and unjustified.

A systems model for solving problems

A system is something which has a number of elements which together make a whole. It is potentially efficient, reliable, replicable and purposeful.

The model presented is adapted from the Bailey–Claus systems model and provides the nurse with a step-by-step approach to making decisions and accounting for them.

Adaptation of Bailey – Claus system model diagram

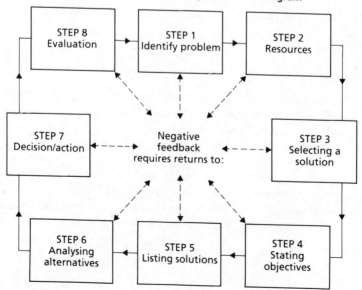

> *A problem is defined as a discrepancy which exists*
> *between what actually is, and what should or could be*

In order to identify the problem, accurate information is required.
A clear statement of what *should* be, must be made.
The exact nature of the discrepancy must be pinpointed.
Symptoms which could account for the discrepancy should be
itemized.

> *The decision maker must review the resources*
> *that are available to solve the problem*

Resources may be material or human.
Material resources include such things as equipment, finances, space,
buildings or time.
The quality and quantity of the health care team must be considered.
Patients/clients should be included in the review as they may have a
significant contribution to make.
Relatives and visitors are important resources, and could affect, or be
affected by any changes which occur.

> *A framework or model for problem-solving*
> *must be selected*

It is important to note that there are various approaches, so that if one
fails, another framework may be more appropriate.
Approaches to problem-solving include:
- focusing on a specific objective, or on immediate relief of
pressure.
- searching for the first acceptable, workable solution.
- finding the best possible alternative course of action.
Some decisions have to be made which are difficult to retract, and may
not allow for feedback: for example, staff appointments.

> *Nurses must be able to state precisely*
> *what they want to accomplish*

Objectives should be stated. These are the expected outcomes, which are phrased in observable performance terms.

A time limit for the outcome may be imposed by the objectives.

All objectives stated will have some influence on the course of action selected.

Objectives should be listed in order of priority.

Objectives can be classified as:

- *critical*, that is those for which an alternative action is unacceptable. For example, if the objective is to alleviate pain, any alternative which does not relieve pain is unacceptable.
- *non-critical*, that is those which are desirable but may be concerned with the decision maker's value system, and may therefore prove unsatisfactory. For example, a non-smoking nurse may tell a patient that he should stop smoking immediately, or he will damage his health. However, the patient may choose to ignore this advice.

> *A variety of solutions may be found*

Using past experience and knowledge, categorizing and utilizing all available information may help to generate alternative solutions.

Nurses must apply creative skills to the problem-solving process.

Evaluation of resources should be carried out so that acceptable and effective alternatives can be recognized.

The advice, and expertise of others should be obtained. This may best be achieved by forming a designated problem-solving committee.

The alternatives must be analysed

Having listed alternative solutions each should be tested against the objectives determined earlier.

Each alternative should be tested against each objective, and if it fails, should be rejected.

Undesirable consequences and side effects should be taken into consideration.

A course of action must be chosen and implemented

One or more persons should be designated to carry out the actions identified.

Follow-up directives to staff members may need to be formulated.

Reporting procedures should be established so that progress can be followed.

Specific reporting dates must be set so that action can be systematically evaluated.

A warning system should be established to indicate if the decision is leading to difficulties.

The outcome must be monitored.

The effectiveness of decision making should be evaluated

Formal evaluation consists of comparing observable performance with objectives determined at the outset.

Positive feedback indicates that the correct decisions were taken.

Negative feedback indicates that the decision/action taken did not solve the problem adequately:

- corrective action can be taken by recycling the decision through the sequence, beginning at any point where a difficulty is evident.

Further reading

Bailey J.T. & Claus K.E. (1975) *Decision Making in Nursing,* Ch. 2–3. C.V. Mosby.

A Systematic Approach to Patient Care: An Introduction. Open University Press, Milton Keynes.

Decision making

Steps	Problem 1	Problem 2	Problem 3
1 Identify the problem	A trained nurse has telephoned to say she is ill and will not be on duty	An elderly male patient admitted the previous day with a CVA has become incontinent	A patient is lying in a soiled bed. There is no clean bed. There is no clean linen in the cupboard
2 Resources	1 trained nurse, 2 students, 1 auxiliary for 20 patients, 15 of whom are very ill and dependent	Catheter Inco-pad/bottle Penile sheath Incontinence advisor	Hospital linen store Another ward linen store Hospital Administration Disposable sheets
3 Selecting a solution	Focus on a specific objective, you need to relieve the pressure!	Search for an acceptable, workable solution	Find the best possible course of action
4 Stating objectives	To manage with fewer staff To give adequate patient care	Manage the incontinence for the patient Aim at independent control as soon as possible	Place the patient in a clean environment

5 Listing solutions	(1) Demand another nurse (2) Ask the nurse to reconsider and come in for part of the day (3) Put problem in writing (4) Ask the night nurse to stay on duty (5) Give priority care only	(1) Catheterize patient (2) Prop a urinal in the bed (3) Put on a penile sheath (4) Consult the incontinence advisor	(1) Turn the sheet over (2) Use disposable sheets (3) Request extra supplies from linen store (4) Increase the linen inventory
6 Analysing alternatives	(1) Another nurse might not be available (2) This is unacceptable pressurization (3) This must be documented (4) It would not be safe to do this (5) The best solution	(1) The doctor must do this but it should only be done when all else fails (2) This might be knocked over causing distress and pressure damage (3) This is a reasonable solution (4) This is probably the best solution	(1) This is unthinkable (2) This is only acceptable if all else fails (3) This may achieve results (4) A long term strategy
7 Decision/Action	Give priority care only	Apply a penile sheath and then consult the incontinence advisor as soon as possible	Put disposable sheets on bed as a temporary measure if linen supplies not forthcoming, and discuss inventory needs with linen store
8 Evaluation	Patients safe and comfortable but nurses are tired and unhappy	Incontinence controlled— bed not wet	Bed clean and dry but not comfortable

Nursing Management

Management is a learned process.

All nurses are managers to some degree.

Effective managers must know themselves, and be able to identify their strengths, weaknesses and capacity for growth and development.

They should have a knowledge of management theory, and be able to get the right things done at the right time.

The activities of management can be divided into two main areas, those of:
- a mechanistic/thinking nature
- a dynamic/doing nature

These are represented in the model below (after Lemin, 1978).

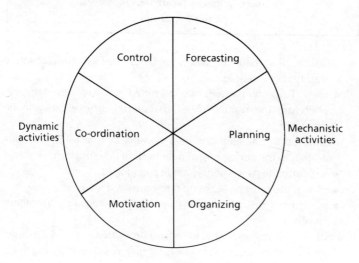

Cycle of management

Each area of activity is of equal importance.

No matter how well the mechanistic activities have been pursued, unless, when the plan is implemented, the dynamic activities are right, problems will arise.

Two other activities must be considered to complete the management function. These are: communication, which binds all the other activities together; and decision making, which forms the basis of management dynamics. (These aspects are considered elsewhere in the text.)

1 Mechanistic activities

> **Forecasting** *can be defined as the analysis*
> *of relevant information from the past, and present,*
> *in order to assess future developments,*
> *and plan ahead*

In nursing, the manager can sometimes forecast with absolute certainty. For example:
- each Tuesday patients are admitted for day case surgery. Therefore the number of staff required to give care can be predicted.

Sometimes the manager can be less sure in forecasting, as, for example, in the appointing of new staff. In this situation:
- look into the past—peruse application forms,
- look at the present—take up references and interview,
- predict the future—trust own judgement, consult with others involved.

It should be remembered that long term prediction involves a greater degree of uncertainty. Therefore higher risks may be involved when planning.

> **Planning** *is determining a course of action*
> *which enables the organization*
> *to meet its stated objectives*

The manager should identify realistic goals.

If the goal is long term, forward planning may be protracted, in order that all the risk factors are identified.

Information which will help in the formulation of the plan should be gathered.

Conclusions should be drawn from all the available data, not isolated parts.

A course of action should be outlined to achieve the goals.

The plan should be simple in concept, clear, objective, easily implemented and controlled, flexible and complete.

Results should be continuously matched against objectives; planning is a dynamic process.

> **Organizing** *ensures that all staff are contributing*
> *to the achievement of the planned goals*
> *of the organization with maximum efficiency*

The manager must identify the work to be completed.

Work must be allocated to appropriately qualified and experienced persons.

There should be a minimum overlap of work commitments.

The manager should pace and support the work, making resources available at the right time and in the right place.

Progress should be checked, but in an acceptable manner.

2 Dynamic activities

The manager must motivate, co-ordinate, and control staff, working with, and through them, for effective results.

Human behaviour is seldom random in nature. It is usually directed toward specific goals.

> **Motivation** *involves creating a climate*
> *in which the employee wants to work*

Personal motivation on the part of the manager may encourage flexible, creative and rational behaviour in others.

Allowing staff to assume responsibility for certain areas of work may assist motivation.

The manager should ensure adequate opportunities for staff to experience a sense of achievement.

Opportunities should be created for growth and advancement.

Staff should be given recognition for work they have undertaken.

> **Co-ordination** *is achieved by maintaining a balanced team and ensuring suitable allocation of work activities, this should lead to team harmony*

The manager's attendance at policy making meetings may be of assistance in the overall co-ordination of work.

A planning scheme should be produced and made available to all team members.

Management responsibilities, and those of the team, should be defined.

Effective communication networks should be established.

The manager should have daily contact with the team.

Team meetings should be held at regular intervals.

Any personality problems likely to arise should be identified; undiagnosed and uncorrected these may lead to team difficulties. Time, counselling, and leading by example may resolve the situation.

> *In the process of* **control** *the manager formulates his intention, ensures action through another, and receives information that his instructions have been fulfilled*

The concept of control is implicit in an organization such as the Health Service which monitors the activities of the workforce.

The manager must decide what is to be achieved in terms of personal or organizational objectives. This requires a yardstick of quality or quantity to serve as a standard.

Current performance must be measured in relation to the achievement required. Information about performance must be received at the appropriate time for effective action.

Corrective action to ensure that objectives are met may involve enabling the employee to exercise control over his own performance, or compelling change in behaviour.

Further reading

Holle M.L. & Blatchley M.E. (1982) *Introduction to Leadership and Management in Nursing*. Wandsworth Health Services Division. Monterey, California.
Lemin B. (1978) *First Line Nursing Management*. Pitman Medical, London.
Schurr M. (1975) *Nurse and Management*. English Universities Press, London.
Stapleton M.E. (1983) *Ward Sisters—Another Perspective*. Royal College of Nurses, London.

Nursing Research

Research has been defined as a systematic investigation aimed at increasing the sum of knowledge.

Nursing research investigates those aspects of professional activity that are predominantly, or appropriately, the concern and responsibility of the nurse.

Research may arise out of theory, but also leads to the development of new theory.

Pure or basic research produces knowledge for the sake of knowledge, and can be said to produce theories *of* nursing.

Applied research may determine the direction of change, solve specific problems, assist in decision making, or in the development or evaluation of nursing practices or products. It also provides theories *for* nursing.

Innovation in clinical practice, and in the education of nurses must be based on the sure foundation of a sound body of knowledge, refined through research. Nursing research not only facilitates the development of improvements in patient care, but also places nursing in an independent position regarding the knowledge from which professional decisions are made.

In the current climate of nursing there is a need for all to develop 'research mindedness'—a critical, questioning, open approach to work, and for some to initiate actual research projects.

The first step in the research process is to identify an area of interest, which can sustain the motivation of the researcher for the period of time it takes to complete the project. Research questions may arise from personal interests or from unresolved problems in professional practice. Once the broad topic area has been identified, exploratory work must be undertaken in order to critically define the research topic.

> *The literature review is an essential component*
> *of the research process*

The review gives in-depth knowledge in a specific topic area.

It may confirm the existence of a problem, and clarify the purpose of the study.

It assists the researcher in the formulation of the plan/proposal.

A method and suitable measuring devices may be identified from the review.

The review can be used to guide all phases of the work.

It aids in relating the outcomes of the study to other findings, providing useful comparative data when results are analysed.

Findings from the review may lead to a need to redefine the problem or have an effect on the research design.

> *The problem selected should be stated*
> *in concise, specific, and testable terms*

The statement of the problem gives an unequivocal set of criteria by
which to judge research planning decisions.

Ideally, in nursing, the problem should be derived from study of
experience, nursing theory or a related discipline theory.

The problem *may* be formulated in the form of an hypothesis—this is
an untested proposition, and is a useful and practical way of
signalling the intentions of the researcher to others.

> *A research design should be chosen which is appropriate*
> *to the problem and purpose of the study*

The way in which the research question has been conceptualized may
indicate the most appropriate design.

Other factors which may need to be taken into consideration include
such things as time, financial constraints, or the setting to be used.

The design enables the researcher to find the answer to the particular
question asked.

Research may be:
- *qualitative*, in which the nature or behaviour of things, or people,
  are examined and tested in an analytical, or speculative way.
- *quantitative*, in which aspects of people or things are measured
  by means of statistical techniques.

Historical, descriptive, experimental or action research approaches
may be adopted.

The design should include:
- a definition of relevant concepts, constructs, and operational
  terms used.
- a description of the setting for the work.
- an outline of the method of data collection, detailed enough to
  allow replication of the work by others.
- a description of the procedures to be used to analyse the data.
- a rationale for the selection of data sources.

A well written proposal is essential if funding is required, or specialist
services and support are to be requested.

> *It is customary and wise to carry out a pilot study*
> *i.e. the plan in miniature*

The pilot study may help to determine the feasibility of conducting a major study.

It should verify the adequacy of the researcher's conceptualization.

Problems in research design may be highlighted, and an opportunity afforded for revision.

It may allow refinement of measuring instruments, and verify the viability of analytical procedures.

It gives the researcher small-scale experience with subjects, methods and instruments.

> *Accurate data collection and analysis will allow*
> *valid conclusions to be drawn*

A variety of techniques will be used for data collection dependent on the research approach.

There should be a sound rationale for the procedures selected, and a reasonable attempt to ensure reliability and validity.

As much data as is reasonable should be collected, weighing it for value, relevance and practical application to the research question.

Where the subject of the research is a person, informed consent to collect data must be obtained.

The person should be given adequate information of the specific action required of him whilst actually involved in the data collection process.

The researcher is bound to maintain confidentiality regarding data, as it pertains to specific individuals.

Efforts should be made to minimize any negative effects on the individual or the environment.

It is critical that the person analysing the data has the necessary skills for the purpose. Help should be sought when required.

Statistical analysis of data provides methods of assessing the validity of the evidence in relation to the problem identified, and a guide for deciding whether or not to reject the original hypothesis.

Positive findings support the hypothesis, or demonstrate trends in a predicted direction.

Negative findings, providing they are not due to poor methodology, are also important, and should be declared accurately and honestly.

Findings may support the general body of knowledge in a given area.

Results may support hitherto suspected, but not proven ideas, thus contributing to the advancement of knowledge.

The findings may contribute entirely new knowledge.

A theory may be reinforced or weakened by the findings.

Serendipity—in the course of the work, completely unexpected findings may be encountered, which may or may not be related to the research. This may need to be reported, and may, indeed, form the basis for subsequent research.

Recommendations from the study may include the implications of the findings for nursing practice, the educational implications, and the need for replication of the study, or additional research in the area.

The findings should be communicated to all who assisted in the implementation of the research.

The project should be written up objectively, clearly and as succinctly as possible, without losing important information.

A concise abstract may be of use in helping the reader to identify the purpose of the work, the methodology employed, the findings, and the conclusions drawn.

Further reading

Calman J. (1976) *One way to do Research*. W. Heinemann Medical Books Ltd, London.

Castle W.M. (1972) *Statistics in Small Doses*. Churchill Livingstone, London.

Krampitz S.D. & Pavlovich N. *Reading for Nursing Research*, C.V. Mosby Co. St Louis, Missouri.

Macleod-Clarke J. & Stodulski A. (1978) How to find out: A guide for searching the nursing literature. *Nursing Times* **74**(b) Occasional paper.

Moroney M.J. (1965) *Facts from Figures*. Penguin, Harmondsworth. (An introduction to statistics.)

Teaching

Teaching is a system of actions intended to bring about or encourage learning.

Learning is the ability to acquire new patterns of behaviour and to modify responses to situations, which should persist, and be retained over a period of time.

> *Teaching can occur both informally and formally within the work setting*

Informal teaching may result from the nurse acting as a role model to others around her. It must be remembered that behaviours reflect attitudes as well as other skills.

Informal teaching can also arise as the nurse is going about her duties. For example, learning can occur during casual conversation, when giving advice or suggestions, or when carrying out some observed nursing practice.

Even if teaching is informal, it should, if possible, be integrated into an overall teaching plan.

Formal teaching involves the planning of a strategy to meet learning needs.

> *The teacher must be clear to whom the teaching is addressed*

Is the learner a patient/client, or relative?

Is the learner a member of the nursing profession?

Is the learner a child or an adult, male or female?

Is the learner of normal intelligence or slow in learning?

Is the learner ill or well?

The content of the session, the level of knowledge to aim for, and the pace of the session may be determined by the answers to these questions.

> *There are two main criteria to consider when deciding the teaching topic*

What the learner wants or needs to know should be taken into account.

What the teacher is able or willing to teach should be identified.

Before any planning is undertaken both criteria should be addressed.

> *Choosing the right location for the teaching session is important in order that effective learning takes place*

The size of the room should be considered. This will depend on the size of the group, any group activities which may take place, and the availability of the room for the length of time required.

Distractions, which might disturb the session, for example people passing through, or noise levels, should be kept to a minimum.

Lighting and ventilation should be adjusted for comfort.

Seating and the need to see what is happening, both for the learner and the teacher, should be borne in mind.

The need for privacy should be considered.

> *The most appropriate time for teaching must be identified*

The optimum time for learning is the first half of the morning, but this is not always possible or achievable.

Motivation to learn is important. This can overcome tiredness after a busy day, or lassitude perhaps after a meal.

A well planned short session, with built in rest times, may promote effective learning. (NB the attention span for a healthy adult is approximately 20 minutes.)

Variation in teaching method may sustain interest and promote learning.

> *The aim or purpose of the session should be agreed between the learner and the teacher*

Agreement will enable the teacher to set learning objectives which are realistic and achievable for both partners.

In setting clear objectives, evaluation of the session is made possible.

> *There are a variety of ways in which*
> *teaching and learning are facilitated*

Sufficient time for preparation should be allowed in order to be confident during presentation.

Reading around the topic leads to a broader knowledge base for the teacher, thus aiding confidence and ability.

Preparation of the room, and the equipment reduces the risk of disturbance during the session.

Selection of appropriate audio-visual aids adds interest to a session.

Selection of an appropriate teaching method with which both the learner and teacher feel secure, aids learning.

At the end of any teaching session, the teacher and learner should ascertain that learning objectives have been achieved. This may come from direct feedback, or observed change in behaviour over a period of time.

Using the six principles in planning teaching

	Plan 1	Plan 2	Plan 3
Who	Mr X, aged 33 years. Newly diagnosed with diabetes mellitus	Three first year student nurses	Miss X, a 58-year old school teacher whose mother has an indwelling catheter
What	The method of insulin administration	To transfer a patient into the bath using a mechanical hoist	1 The principles of asepsis 2 The method of changing a catheter bag
Where	Treatment room	Bathroom	Bedside
When	Twice daily at normal times of administration, until patient feels confident	When desired by the patient	During evening visits until daughter feels confident
Why	To enable him to administer his own insulin on discharge home	To enable students to use a hoist safely to transfer a patient	To ensure daughter understands principles of catheter care in order to care for mother at home
How	1 Demonstration 2 Practice under supervision using a facsimile 3 Self injection under supervision	1 Demonstration of equipment and how it is used to place patient in bath 2 Students transferred on hoist— experiential learning 3 Assisted practice 4 Supervised practice	Demonstration followed by supervised practice

Preparation	1 A clear work surface provided 2 Privacy ensured 3 All equipment available	1 Discuss principles of hoists 2 Ensure hoist in working order 3 Prepare bath, bathroom, etc. 4 Discuss learning exercise with patient, gaining consent	1 Collect all equipment 2 Allow adequate time for teaching
Evaluation	Patient can inject himself safely	Patient comfortable and safely transferred	Bag changed safely, mother and daughter satisfied

Further reading

Jarvis P. (1983) *Professional Education*. Croom Helm Ltd, Beckenham.
Rogers T (1977) *Adults Learning*, 2nd edition. Open University Press, Milton Keynes.
Wilson-Barnett J. (1983) *Patient Teaching*. Churchill Livingstone, Edinburgh.

Index